ROSEMARY CONLEY'S WHOLE BODY PROGRAMME

Rosemary Conley lives in Leicestershire with her husband and business partner, Mike Rimmington, with whom she runs Rosemary Conley Enterprises.

A qualified exercise teacher, Rosemary has worked in the field of slimming and exercise for twenty years, but it was in 1986 that she discovered by accident that low-fat eating led to a leaner body. Forced on to a very low-fat diet as a result of a gallstone problem, not only did Rosemary avoid surgery, but her previously disproportionately large hips and thighs reduced dramatically in size. After extensive research and trials her *Hip and Thigh Diet* was published in 1988 by Arrow Books. This book and its sequel, *Rosemary Conley's Complete Hip and Thigh Diet*, have dominated the paperback bestseller lists for over three years and have sold in excess of 2 million copies. *Rosemary Conley's Hip and Thigh Diet* has been translated into five languages including Hebrew and Greek.

Subsequently, her *Hip and Thigh Diet Cookbook, Inch Loss Plan* and *Metabolism Booster Diet* have also been instant Number 1 bestsellers and Rosemary has been accepted as the leading authority in the United Kingdom on weight and inch loss.

In 1990 Rosemary was given her own series on network BBC 1 television. Her brief was to encourage the nation to exercise and adopt a healthy, low fat diet. Her *Diet and Fitness Club Action Pack* (BBC Books) which accompanied the series was yet another bestseller. The series is to be continued in 1992.

In 1991 her *Whole Body Programme* video was launched by BBC Video. It too became a Number 1 bestseller, topping the UK video charts for many months, and is, to date, the bestselling fitness video to have been released in this country. Rosemary was awarded a Triple Platinum Award for sales exceeding 300,000 copies.

When asked why she has enjoyed so much success, she says: 'It's simply because my diets and exercises work for ordinary, real people.'

Rosemary is a committed Christian, and has a daughter, Dawn, by her first marriage.

Also in Arrow by Rosemary Conley
Rosemary Conley's Hip and Thigh Diet
Rosemary Conley's Complete Hip and Thigh Diet
Rosemary Conley's Hip and Thigh Diet Cookbook
Rosemary Conley's Inch Loss Plan
Rosemary Conley's Metabolism Booster Diet

ROSEMARY CONLEY'S
WHOLE BODY
PROGRAMME

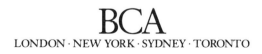
BCA
LONDON · NEW YORK · SYDNEY · TORONTO

This edition published in 1992 by
BCA
by arrangement with Arrow Books

CN 1970

Typeset by SX Composing Ltd, Rayleigh, Essex
Printed and bound in Great Britain by
Butler & Tanner Ltd, Frome and London

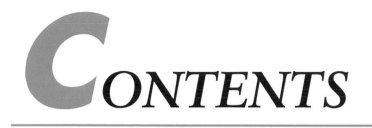ONTENTS

ACKNOWLEDGEMENTS

With the increasing pressures placed upon my time, and the ever decreasing amount of time in which to write my books, I find myself even more greatly indebted to my family and colleagues as another book is completed. Without their support, help and co-operation this book would not have been written.

I would like to acknowledge the intense hard work of my editor Jan Bowmer at Arrow and the copy editor Valerie Buckingham who tirelessly ploughed through the complicated copy as it arrived, via the fax machine, in disjointed batches hot off the wordprocessor! Special thanks also to Sara Kidd, who so painstakingly worked through the endless number of photographs and who has designed this book so attractively. Special thanks also to Dennis Barker at Arrow for the cover design and to Suzanne Webber and Frank Phillips at BBC Books. There are also numerous others who worked so assiduously to produce this book in time. Thank you all so much.

I would also like to thank Roselyne Masselin for contributing the Vegetarian chapter, Jane Ashton for her help in the Pregnancy chapter, and Kim Hames and Patricia Bourne for a number of the recipes.

Thanks also must go to my daughter Dawn for typing so much of the manuscript for me, and also my secretary, Diane Stevens. I would also like to thank my husband, Mike, for his patience and support during the writing of this book and also the support of our special friends Stephen, Wendy, Ian and Ruth. Thank you all very much indeed.

INTRODUCTION

Would you like to feel proud of your body instead of wanting to hide it? Would you like to radiate youthfulness, vitality and health rather than remain overweight, unhealthy, unfit and uninspired?

For twenty years now, I have been in the business of helping people to lose weight, and over the last six years I have actively researched the needs and desires of dieters across the world who have witnessed the extraordinary effectiveness of my low-fat diets on their bodies. In addition, I am constantly aware of *my own* war against fat. It is because of my continuing determination to win this war, not just for myself but for others too who wish to improve their health, fitness and self-esteem, that I have written this book. In devising a plan which combines diet and exercise in the most effective way to reduce fat and improve our body shape, I have tried to cater for every practical and social need. This book contains what I believe to be the ultimate weight and inch loss plan – THE WHOLE BODY PROGRAMME.

Since my original *Hip and Thigh Diet* was published in 1988, I have received many thousands of letters from readers who have achieved dieting success as a result of following one of my diet plans. In previous books I included many extracts from these letters in the hope that prospective dieters would be encourged by those successes. Many wrote to say it was these testimonials that made them decide to give the diet a try. It is impossible to include them here, but I feel the following letter from Marina Escott will help to encourage and inspire a great number of people in all age groups. Marina wrote:

'I wrote to you a little while back to tell you how thrilled I am with your video and books. With their help, my hubby and I have lost weight so easily.

'I thought you would be interested to know that I have had a weight problem ALL my life; in my younger years I was actually 17 st 3 lbs (109.2kg), a fact I feel ashamed to admit. To cut a very long story short, I dieted, joined clubs and lost around 2–3 st (12.7-19kg), only to pile the pounds back on as soon as I stopped dieting. As you can imagine, all the loose ugly skin at the tops of my legs, and especially around my middle, caused me much distress, to say the least. My hubby and my daughter often said I would never get rid of the loose skin unless I had an operation. Well, Rosemary, I am thrilled to be able to tell you it has gone! My family can't believe their eyes. It's entirely due to the exercises in your Whole Body Programme video which I practise nearly every day, including weekends and holidays. I even take an audio cassette of the exercises when we go away to our caravan, so I can still practise them to music. I take my mat and do the exercises on the patio (outside the caravan), with neighbours and anyone else looking on and pulling my leg, but to no avail. I just shout, "Come and join me!"

'People say how slim I look and it's all thanks to your sensible low-fat eating plan and exercises. Believe me, to actually see all my unsightly skin disappearing before my very eyes is enough to make me continue with the exercises. After all, when people ask how I spare the time, I am absolutely speechless and say, "Goodness, what's 50 *minutes a day!" If I can do it, anyone can, and my work and home do not suffer because of it. I benefit from feeling so well. I tell all my friends I feel better now at 56 years of age than I did when I was 30. My husband agrees wholeheartedly and says I look better too!*

'I am looking forward to your new release, and I hope my story may inspire other women of my age-group.'

At the end of my Diet and Fitness television series last year, we invited some of the viewers to join me and speak of their success on the diet. Here are some of those who appeared.

PHIL AND JULIE JUKES

Julie was only 16 and weighed around 9 st (57.1kg) when she met 17-year-old Phil Jukes. Twelve months later they were married. Julie said: 'Phil only weighed 8 st (50.8kg) on our wedding day. He was actually quite thin because he is 5 ft 10 ins (1.8m) tall.'

Julie's superb cooking together with their habit of snacking on crisps and sweets led to them both gaining weight. Six years later Julie was expecting their first child. Her weight increased to 11½ st (69.8kg), but shortly after Robert was born she did lose some weight and went down to around 10½ st (72.9kg). Despite being only 5ft 3ins (1.6m) tall, she didn't feel particularly overweight. Two years later Julie was pregnant again but this time she ballooned to a mighty 16 st (101.6kg). She knew she was eating a lot but she felt unable to control it. Eight weeks after Mitchel was born Julie decided to make a concerted effort to diet. Her sister-in-law had successfully lost 2 st (12.7kg) on my Complete Hip and Thigh Diet and Julie decided to try it too. She hated herself for being so overweight and was determined to succeed. She went back to work in the evenings when Mitchel was 8 weeks old and she says this helped her to cope with the diet. While she was at work she was away from food and temptation. In a matter of a few months Julie lost 3½ st (22.6kg).

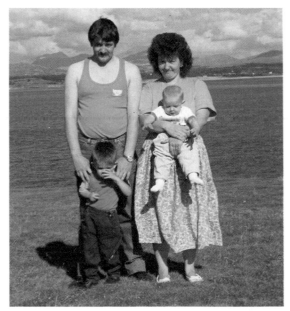
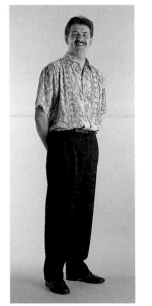
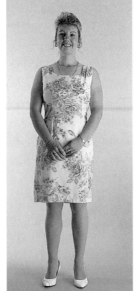

BEFORE   AFTER

She suggested Phil join her in her dieting campaign, as he was now significantly heavier than when they first met. They weighed in on the high street chemist's scales and Phil was quite shocked to find he weighed almost 13 st (82.5kg). He immediately embarked on the diet and lost his excess 2 st (12.7kg) in just 8 weeks. 'Phil was so strict while he was on the diet. He didn't falter once and the weight just seemed to drop off him,' said Julie.

Julie continued her slimming campaign, this time with my Metabolism Booster Diet, and lost another 2½ st (15.8kg), making a total loss of 6 st (38.1kg) in 14 months. She and Phil were thrilled.

Phil keeps fit by playing football three times a week and Julie attends two keep fit classes a week and also swims regularly and cycles to work. They say they both feel fitter and better than ever. Julie added: 'I never felt hungry, except first thing in the morning. I found both diets very enjoyable and easy to follow. I feel wonderful now I have lost all that fat. I hope I look as wonderful as I feel.' Well, you certainly do, Julie!

Phil didn't record his inch losses but Julie lost 9 ins (23cm) from her bust, 17 ins (43.1cm) from her waist, 13½ ins (34.2cm) from her hips, 12½ ins (37.1cm) from her widest part, almost 6ins (15.2cm) from each thigh and almost 5ins (12.7cm) from each knee.

COLLETTE BECKETT

Collette is just 5 ft 2 ins (1.57m) and weighed almost 10½ st (72.9kg) when she decided to go on my diet.

She said:

'I always believed my big thighs and hips were due to my frame size and, no matter how much weight I lost, they would always remain large. But your low-fat diet proved me wrong. My legs are nice and slim now and I think the exercises helped enormously. Now, if I've had a bad day and have eaten a lot, all I have to do is follow the Whole Body Programme video and be a bit careful the next day about what I eat. Now my weight seems to remain more or less constant even though I'm not so strict with food. Everyone told me that because I'd lost weight so quickly, it would come back quickly and I'd end up heavier than before. Those people are still eating their words. I've stayed this slim for about five months now.'

Collette lost 2½ st (15.8kg) in 8 weeks. In that time she lost 2 ins (5cm) from her bust, 3 ins (8cm) from her waist, 4 ins (10cm) from her hips and 5 ins (12.7cm) from her widest part. Her thighs have reduced to a very slim 18 ins (45cm) each and her vital statistics are an enviable 34-23-33 ins (86-60-83cm).

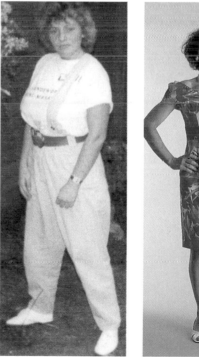

BEFORE   **AFTER**

TRACEY BRYAN

Tracey Bryan lost 2 st 9 lbs (16.7kg) in 14 weeks on my low-fat diet. She is now a delightfully slim 9 st 12 lbs (62.5kg), ideal for her 5 ft 7½ ins (1.7m) height.

Tracey said:

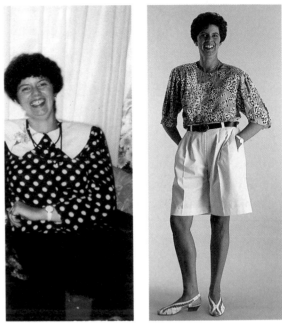

BEFORE   AFTER

'*I started your diet in January with friends from my little girl's toddlers group. Since then I have gone past my goal weight of 10 st 7 lbs (72.9kg). I am now 9 st 12 lbs (62.5 kg) and I have never felt better. I have just returned from holiday and I was able to join in all the sports as I felt so much fitter.*

'*I think, in addition to the diet, the exercises from your Whole Body Programme video were a great help too. I would recommend this diet and exercise programme to anyone.*'

WEIGHTS AND MEASURES

The following conversion rates have been used throughout this book:

1 oz = 25g   1 fl oz = 25ml   ½ pint = 250ml

HEALTH WARNING

In the interest of good health it is always important to consult your doctor before commencing any diet or exercise programme.

HOW TO LOSE THE MAXIMUM WEIGHT IN THE MINIMUM TIME

There is an art to losing unwanted weight healthily and to losing it in the shortest possible time. But there is no magic formula. We have to take into account the various factors affecting our age and our everyday lifestyle, as well as our current physical condition. We also need to understand exactly *how* we can achieve a better figure. It very definitely is not just a matter of weighing less on the scales.

Our body is a remarkable piece of construction comprising a mass of organs, muscles, bones, tissues and blood, all ingeniously worked in together to form an incredibly powerful machine. If well maintained and not overloaded it can last around a hundred years. Just as a motor car that is lovingly driven, maintained and cleaned can look wonderful even when getting on in years, so too can *our* body.

There are two very important elements that come into play in attempting to achieve a leaner and healthier body. In broad terms it is what we eat that determines how fat we are, and it is the physical exercise we undertake that determines our muscle tone and our level of fitness. Many people believe that they cannot lose weight without exercising. This is absolutely not the case.

Before we even consider how we can speed up our rate of weight loss it is essential to understand how our body uses its intake of calories which it receives regularly in the form of food and drink.

What is metabolism?

Anyone interested in losing weight will almost certainly have heard the word metabolism. Our metabolism is the mechanism within our body that effects a chemical breakdown of the foods we eat and results in the utilisation of the nutrients the body needs to carry out repairs, renewal and growth as well as to generate the energy we need to cope with our everyday activities.

What about calories?

Our metabolic rate is the rate at which our body burns up calories. A calorie is a unit of heat and that heat provides energy. The more energy we expend, the hotter we become and the more calories we burn up. This is where exercise can help to accelerate weight loss. However, the majority of our calories are automatically utilised by the body to renew and repair body tissue, to grow our hair and nails, and to provide enough energy to pump blood around the body through the heart to supply all the oxygen we need via our lungs, non-stop throughout our entire life. The amount of energy (calories) our body needs for these functions alone is determined by our individual basal metabolic rate (b.m.r.). The average basal metabolic rate of a woman is about 1400 calories per day and for a man it is approximately 1800. The basal metabolic rate can be increased by regular physical activity. Generally speaking, the average b.m.r. of men is subject to greater variance than that of women, proportionate to the degree of physical activity involved in their everyday work. The b.m.r. can also be reduced, not by lack of exercise, but by a reduced calorie intake. If the body receives insufficient calories to supply its physiological needs the b.m.r. will reduce to a level that will still fulfil the body's basic requirements. This is exactly the opposite of what the slimmer wants to happen. It is therefore essential for dieters to keep their b.m.r. as high as possible by eating sufficient calories – around 1400–1500 calories for women and 1800–1900 calories for men.

It is easy to lose weight on this intake of calories because from the moment we get out of bed in the morning we start (and continue) to use calories in addition to those used by our b.m.r. for bodily functions. The extra energy we *need* will be supplied from the excess fat stored on our body. This principle forms the basis of any weight-reducing diet.

Are all calories the same?

Recent clinical studies have examined the effect on the body of fat calories compared with that of carbohydrate calories. Obviously our calorie intake has to be controlled if we are to lose weight. However, research has concluded that we can eat proportionately more carbohydrate calories than fat calories and in fact lose more weight. This is why low-fat diets work so efficiently and why so

many followers of my diets have said that the most important contributory factor to their success was the large amount of food they were allowed to eat. We can eat more food on a low-fat diet because, ounce for ounce, or gram for gram, carbohydrates contain half the calories of fats. It is for this reason that I allow my dieters to consume unlimited amounts of potatoes with their main meal of the day.

And what about exercise?

To encourage maximum weight loss we can increase our physical activity so that we burn even more calories. Just as a motor car burns up more fuel when it goes faster, so will our body. And the bonus of increased physical exercise is an increase in our b.m.r! So, we can lose weight by eating just sufficient calories to maintain our b.m.r. and to enable the body to function properly. Then simply going about our everyday tasks will cause our body to go into energy deficit. If we don't give our body extra fuel (food) to supply that increased need, it will call on its reserve supplies – *fat*. However, if we INCREASE that energy deficit by being MORE physically active than usual, we can lose even *more* fat.

Do I have to count calories?

By way of explanation I have discussed calorie counting here, but readers of my earlier books will be very much aware of my distaste for the negative habit of counting anything to do with food, whether it be units, grams or calories. It's all very well, but what happens when you run out of your daily allowance by 4pm? Inevitably, the prospect of an evening of starvation can lead to an almighty eating binge. Result: diet abandoned and weight GAIN instead of weight loss.

When I design my diets I do roughly count the number of calories. Some menus contain more calories than others but as long as you vary the choice of meals, any difference will balance out.

So what can I eat?

I believe it is important to have a certain amount of freedom on a diet and for this reason I allow unlimited quantities of vegetables to be served with the main meal of the day. Vegetables are extremely useful as a filler. Not only are they economical in terms of calories, they are relatively inexpensive too, particularly if purchased from a market. Vegetables such as carrots, onions, mushrooms, broccoli, spinach, cabbage, Brussels sprouts, courgettes, tomatoes and peppers all contain very few calories (approximately 5 calories per ounce (25g). Peas and sweetcorn contain more, at about 15 calories per ounce (25g), but even so their content is still very low compared with that for poultry, meat, eggs and cheese, which ranges from 50–100 calories per ounce (25g), or the dreaded fat at 220 calories per ounce (25g)! Vegetables can be eaten in simple form or they can be combined in a gastronomic creation to enhance any dinner menu. Follow the suggestions in the recipe sections of this book, or create your own, adapting traditional favourite recipes by eliminating any fat from their preparation.

As I recommend that my dieters should feel full when they leave the dinner table, what better way to fill up than by eating some extra vegetables.

But what about potatoes?

Potatoes are a real friend of the low-fat dieter. They are easy to prepare and in the recipe section you will find details of how to cook oven chips, creamed and roast potatoes, jacket potatoes and a delicious potato and onion bake.

Not only are potatoes relatively low in calories they are also good psychologically. Regarded as totally non-diet-like food, they are considered a bonus in any weight-reducing plan. Years ago we were advised to cut down on bread and potatoes

if we wanted to lose weight. Of course, such a suggestion is now considered absurd. In reality it wasn't the bread or the potatoes that were the culprits. It was the fat we added to them in the form of butter or milk that really did the damage!

I do not limit the consumption of potatoes on my diet. If piling your plate with an extra 3 or 4 ounces (75–100g) of potatoes enables you to feel sufficiently full and satisfied you are far less likely to binge or nibble between meals.

So are all carbohydrates good for us?

Carbohydrates are described as 'good' or 'bad' according to their nutritional value. Foods such as bread, potatoes, rice, pasta and cereal offer a variety of valuable nutrients as well as energy and are termed 'good', whereas 'bad' carbohydrates include foods such as sugar, jam, confectionery and alcohol. These offer little or no nutritional benefit – only empty calories. However, they are included in moderation on my diets for convenience and palatability in the absence of high-fat foods.

Are 'good' carbohydrates low in calories?

Potatoes are low in calories compared with the other 'good' carbohydrates. Old potatoes have 25 calories per ounce (25g). A generous portion would be 4–6 oz (100–150g), amounting to only 100–150 calories. Uncooked rice, however, contains 100 calories per ounce (25g), an average small portion of 2 oz (50g) would therefore total 200 calories; and pasta (uncooked) is 80 calories per ounce (25g), an average 2 oz (50g) portion would yield 160 calories. Pasta and rice should therefore be eaten in some moderation. Women should restrict portions of these to approximately 2 oz (50g) [dry weight] per serving. Men, however, can eat them more freely according to their appetite, since they need the extra calories. Cereal too should be eaten in moderation. An average portion would be 1 oz (25g), generating 100 calories.

But what if I still feel hungry?

If you are to get slim and stay slim you MUST break the habit of eating between meals. It is from these little nibbles that wholesale binges emerge. Bingeing can do immeasurable damage to our diet. Firstly, we feel a total failure and often decide to abandon the diet. Secondly, our natural reaction after bingeing is to starve the next day. If this is done on a regular basis it will slow down our metabolic rate, making long-term weight loss more difficult. It will also inevitably lead to another binge because we will feel so desperately hungry.

REMEMBER...

- Fill up on vegetables at the main meal of the day
- Only eat fruit at mealtimes (as suggested within the diet menus)
- Do not eat between meals

There may be some who read this and think, 'Fine. I won't eat potatoes, rice or pasta, or if I do, I will eat very little. I want to lose weight FAST!' That's all very well, but you will get hungry. Then you will cheat. Then you might binge. And then you might abandon the diet altogether. It is much wiser to fill up on these low-fat carbohydrate foods that give you energy, satisfy your hunger and leave you with no feeling of deprivation. To emphasise the point further, if you have ever kept a weight-loss record, just add up the pounds (kg) that you have *gained* on these starve-binge occasions. If you deduct those pounds (kg) from your present weight, you'll realise how much lighter you would have been now and soon see the folly of trying to be too strict.

When the scales seem to stick!

Whilst I am not a great fan of scales, much preferring a tape measure or a mirror, they still remain the quickest way to monitor progress. However, there are occasions when the scales seem to stick. This always seems to happen after a week when you think you've been saintly. However, reaching a plateau when dieting is common. It is frustrating and annoying and often occurs for those who cut down on their calories too drastically. As explained earlier, the metabolic rate falls if the calorie intake is too low, so it is essential not to eat less than the number of calories required by your basal metabolic rate.

There are two ways to jolt yourself out of a plateau: firstly, by *increasing* your food intake very slightly and, secondly, by breaking up your diet into more meals. A multi-meal diet will effectively maximise your weight-loss progress. Each time you start up your metabolic engine by eating, your body starts burning up calories in order to digest the food. Providing you don't *exceed* your recommended calorie allowance, these temporary measures will help to burn up more calories and result in increased weight loss. However, once you have jolted your metabolism into action and weight loss is again being achieved, I recommend you return to the 3-meals-a-day principle, which is a more 'normal' and convenient way of eating and in the long term is likely to encourage a healthy level of weight maintenance.

'I'm dieting again!...'

Another nuisance for the dieter is the problem of repeat dieting. Losing weight the first time on a diet is comparatively easy because there is a novelty value in following a different way of eating, often with foods we may not have tried before. Also, in the early stages of a diet we tend to be very strict, sticking rigidly to the diet menus and not cheating in between meals. We are also greatly encouraged by the often substantial weight losses in the first week or two, and this spurs us on towards our ultimate goal. Unfortunately, maintaining our new slimmer figure isn't always easy, and unless small weight gains are nipped in the bud, overweight can return.

Second-time dieting is far less rewarding and infinitely more difficult. There are a variety of reasons for this. The body inevitably becomes acclimatised to the healthier eating habits you learned from the diet that are now hopefully a way of life. Therefore there isn't the same drastic change in foods that you experience first time round and subsequently, the drop in calories will be less. Despite having had numerous 'naughty' indulgences to cause your excess weight to return, I am sure you wouldn't have been eating platefuls of fish and chips, cakes, biscuits and chocolates. Therefore, the dietary transition this time will not be as dramatic. Because you 'know' the diet, you are far more likely to make up your own menus instead of following to the letter the ones described in the diet book. As a result of all this, the weight-loss progress is likely to be slower. So, if you *are* dieting for a second time, make sure you follow these simple rules:

- Reread the diet instructions and follow them strictly (even if you managed to get away with cheating last time!).
- Realise that the best way to ruin a diet is to nibble between meals. And don't be tempted to eat fruit when you feel peckish, just because it's low in fat. Fruit contains calories, and if eaten outside the diet recommendations, it will definitely slow down your progress.
- Do watch the quantities of foods where specified – for example, breakfast cereal, meat, poultry, pasta and rice. Don't guess!
- Look carefully at the labels of products when

you're shopping. Select the brands with the least fat and the fewest calories.
- Use *no* fat in cooking, trim all fat from meat and *never* use margarine, butter or low-fat spread on your bread.
- Try having a low-calorie drink before each mealtime. It will help to satisfy your appetite more quickly when you start eating.

Learning to cope with the difficult times

There are times when we find it impossible to fight off temptation. It happens to every dieter at some stage. Accepting that we *will* have lapses, we need to minimise the likely damage.

In times of weakness or depression it is the *instant* comfort foods that appeal. Depending on whether you have a sweet or savoury tooth, it is the biscuits, cakes, sweets, chocolates and ice cream, or the crisps, peanuts and cheese – or, for some people, all of them – that seem irresistible. Recognise what your weaknesses are and try not to have these foods in the house.

Learn to anticipate the bad times. Many women find premenstrual tension plays havoc with their diet. The craving for something sweet seems uncontrollable. At such times, make sure the refrigerator is stocked up with diet drinks and low-calorie, low-fat yogurts or fromage frais to help keep the damage to a minimum.

Lastly, realise that sometimes we *need* to indulge, but if we *restrict* our indulgences they will do little harm. They just slow down our weight-loss progress.

Without doubt, one of the main reasons for the incredible success enjoyed by followers of my low-fat diets has been the simplicity – foods that are easy to buy, menus that are easy to prepare and diets themselves that are very easy to follow. Perhaps most important of all, my dieters don't feel hungry. I try to select foods that are high in nutrition but low in fat and, whenever possible, foods with maximum volume, thus enabling the dieter to enjoy greatest possible exercise for the jaws. Food that requires a good deal of chewing not only makes us feel we are eating more, but inevitably we eat it more slowly. This allows time for the food to reach the stomach before we finish eating and we then have a much better chance of knowing when we have had enough. In addition, foods that require a lot of chewing also usually take a fair bit of digesting, and if the digestive system has to work harder, it burns up more calories. Conversely, foods such as cakes and chocolate that require minimal mastication are extremely high in calories and fat. They are quick to eat and often don't temper our appetites quickly enough, so we end up eating more!

For those less active

Those who are unable to be at all physically active, such as those confined to a wheelchair, will need to reduce their calorie intake below that of an able-bodied dieter. For all those with physical restrictions, I have included some chair exercises on pages 182-184 which I hope will help burn up a few extra calories to encourage and improve weight loss while also increasing circulation and mobility.

MY TOP TEN TIPS FOR SUCCESSFUL SLIMMING:

- 1 We all work better if we have a goal. So decide on a date or, better still, plan your slimming campaign with a deadline in mind – a special occasion such as a wedding, holiday or celebration. Take one day at a time.
- 2 Get rid of all your excuses as to why diets don't work for you. Diets *will* work, and this one is even easier to follow and will be even more effective than before.
- 3 Create a positive environment and mix with others who are successful dieters.
- 4 Learn to handle the difficult times. We all have them. Don't throw in the towel when the going gets tough.
- 5 Develop the habit of enthusiasm about your new eating plan. See the weight and inches disappear and picture yourself succeeding.
- 6 Get rid of temptation whenever possible. Don't keep food in the house that you find difficult to resist. At functions where a buffet is served, ask your partner to fill your plate for you. *Don't* go to the buffet table yourself unless you feel very strong-willed. Whether dining out or at home, don't have any second helpings, except of vegetables or salads.
- 7 Have no doubts about your success. Persistence is a wonderful quality when you are dieting. Persevere and you will reach your goal.
- 8 Enlist the help of a friend to act as your diet companion to encourage you in your campaign towards a better body.
- 9 Weigh and measure yourself at the same time, every week, in the presence of your diet companion. Scales should be placed on a flat board for greatest accuracy and should not be stored in a bathroom, where they are likely to be affected by damp.
- 10 Many confuse desire with their ability to lose weight. If a friend were to offer you £20,000 if you could lose, say, 2 stones (12.8kg) in 10 weeks, I am quite sure you would lose that weight very easily indeed. So realise that it is your *desire* to be slim, not your ability to lose weight, that really determines your success.

STARTING SLOWLY

DIET

Over the next few weeks I would like to reshape YOUR body because I want you to feel good about yourself, not just this year but hopefully for life. I would like you to feel that this year will see a new you – a slimmer, fitter, more confident you.

I want you to aim for leanness, not thinness, for muscles that are toned, not overdeveloped, and a level of fitness that is healthy, not fanatical.

For this Whole Body Programme I have tried to create a diet and exercise plan that will offer greatest scope for free choice, with maximum effect in terms of weight and inch loss, combined with body toning and increased overall fitness. This programme is not intended as a short-term solution to your current possibly overweight, flabby and unhealthy condition. I hope it will help you towards a long-term leaner, longer, healthier and happier life.

However, if you are to succeed you need to re-educate your kitchen as well as your eating and fitness habits. To this end I have included suggestions for your store cupboard and refrigerator so that you will have the most useful ingredients ready to hand.

If you are to have any hope of enjoying success it is essential that you observe the Forbidden List (see page 29), strictly avoiding these foods during your weight-loss programme. When you have reached your target size and weight you may be able to indulge in some of them occasionally. However, I am confident that your attraction towards fatty foods will naturally reduce, if not

diminish completely. Personally, I never thought I would be able to give up cream or butter but I honestly don't miss them at all now. Many of my low-fat dieters have written to me saying they feel exactly the same – even chocoholics have been cured. There is no doubt that low-fat eating in the long term really does reduce your taste for fatty food. Cooking without fat is easier than you think, and, to help you, later in this section I have listed some utensils I feel are a must in a low-fat kitchen.

I believe it is impractical to ask dieters to throw away all their high-fat foods overnight – though I have to say this would be the ideal. Try to eliminate these foods gradually from the kitchen over the next seven days. For practical and economic reasons I feel it is a good idea to ease your way *towards* low-fat eating.

Let the other family members who do not need to diet, particularly the children, eat up any high-fat hard cheeses, sausages, butter, margarine, cakes and biscuits, and consider carefully whether you wish to replace these foods. Before you buy anything, consider if there is a low-fat or low-sugar variety available.

However, if you have young children, you will have to take into account their specific needs. Children under the age of seven should never be placed on a weight-reducing diet as they need energy to make them grow. Nevertheless, good eating habits can be established in childhood and, ultimately, it makes sense to encourage them to eat healthier, low-fat foods. By re-educating their palate now, not only will you help protect them from heart and weight problems in later life, but they are also more likely to pass on healthy eating habits to their own offspring.

Children under the age of two, or children who do not eat a varied diet, should still be fed whole milk, although semi-skimmed milk is considered acceptable for children from the age of two upwards. Skimmed milk, while fine for adults, is not recommended for children under the age of five because it contains less vitamin A and D than semi-skimmed or whole milk.

In addition, children need foods such as cheese to provide extra calcium, but simply by substituting Edam or cottage cheese in place of high-fat cheddar and by encouraging them to eat lots of yogurts, they will be getting plenty of calcium without unnecessary fat. Whilst children do need lots of energy from their food, it is far better for them to eat those extra calories in the form of fresh fruit, such as bananas, than confectionery and biscuits, and from low-fat crisps in preference to the high-fat varieties. Aim for three meals a day and always discourage between-meal snacking. (See pages 151-154 for delicious ideas for children's healthy packed lunches.)

The next time you go shopping, consider the following categories when making your selection. Items in the **Green** list are virtually fat-free and therefore ideal for everyone, particularly anyone trying to lose weight. Foods in the **Amber** list are moderately low in fat and offer healthy options for the whole family and the occasional treat for those on a diet. The **Red** list contains foods that are high in fat, and these should be kept to a minimum within the family diet. Whilst an occasional treat is acceptable for those not wishing to lose weight, high-fat foods can become addictive and, even if you are slim now, they may well lead to overweight in the future. Preventing a weight problem now is so much easier than trying to cure one later.

GREEN

Alcohol: in moderation (not exceeding 21 units a week for men and 14 units a week for women, see page 28)

Beans, lentils and pulses: any type

Bread: any type without fat (not fried or buttered)

Breakfast cereal: any type, except products with nuts

Cakes: very low-fat

Cheese: cottage cheese, fromage frais, Quark (choose low-fat varieties)

Condiments: any type except tartar sauce (see also **Sauces**)

Crispbreads: rye crispbread, Ryvita

Dressings: oil-free dressings, vinegar, lemon juice; reduced-oil dressings in moderation

Eggs: egg whites can be eaten freely, but only a maximum of two egg yolks a week

Fish (including shellfish): any type of white fish (cod, plaice, halibut, whiting, lemon sole), salmon, tuna in brine, cockles, crab, lobster, mussels, oysters, prawns, shrimps; mackerel in moderation

Flour: any type

Fruit: any type of fresh, frozen or tinned fruit, except ackee, avocado, coconut and olives; dried fruit in moderation

Fruit juices: grape juice, apple juice, unsweetened orange, grapefruit, pineapple and exotic fruit juices – all in moderation

Game: any type, roasted without fat and with all skin removed

Grains: any type (see also **Rice**)

Gravy: made with gravy powder, not granules, unless low-fat varieties of granules are used

Jams and preserves: marmalade, jam, honey, syrup – all in moderation

Meat: lean red meat (twice a week maximum), cooked without fat (see also **Game, Offal, Poultry**)

Meat substitutes: textured vegetable protein, vegeburgers

Milk: skimmed or semi-skimmed (silver top with cream removed can be classed as semi-skimmed)

Nuts: chestnuts only

Offal: any type, in moderation, cooked without fat

Pasta: egg-free and fat-free varieties

Pickles and relishes: any type in moderation

Poultry: chicken, duck, turkey – all cooked without fat and with all skin removed

Prepared meals for slimmers: Boots, Lean Cuisine, Menu Plus, Weight Watchers ranges

Puddings: custard made with skimmed milk; fresh fruit salad, fruit cooked or fresh – served with wine, jelly, low-fat Christmas pudding, meringues, rice pudding made with skimmed milk, low-fat varieties of yogurt

Rice: brown rice, boiled or steamed

Sauces: Barbecue Sauce (see recipe, page 109), apple sauce, cranberry sauce, horseradish, brown sauce, tomato ketchup, mint sauce, oil-free vinaigrette, soy sauce, vinegar, Worcestershire sauce, oil-free salad dressing, yogurt dressing, mustard, yeast extract, white sauces made with skimmed milk and no fat (see also **Condiments**)

Soups: clear and non-cream varieties, home-made or branded products

Soya: low-fat type

Stuffing: made with water

Sugar: any type in moderation; artificial sweeteners

Vegetables: any type (except ackee and avocado), cooked and served without fat

Yogurt: any low-fat varieties; avoid Greek

AMBER

Some people are not what could be considered really overweight, but they have a few excess pounds distributed round their body in places they wish were a little trimmer. Alternatively, they may just acknowledge that their eating habits are far from healthy and have decided now is the time to make a few changes. If you are not looking to make a big reduction in your weight but wish to eat healthily, the foods listed here may be used with, and in addition to, those in the **Green** list.

Biscuits: water biscuits

Cakes: low-fat sponge cakes (such as Swiss roll), Jaffa cakes, scones without butter, buns without cream

Cheese: low-fat cheddar, Edam or Gouda

Condiments: tartar sauce

Dressings: reduced-oil salad dressings (all low-fat brands)

Drinks: low-fat varieties of Horlicks, Ovaltine or drinking chocolate

Eggs: except fried

Fish: kippers, rollmop herrings, eels, herrings, sardines, bloaters, sprats

Jams and preserves: lemon curd in moderation

Meat: sausages if well grilled, bacon grilled, beefburgers grilled

Milk: whole milk with cream removed

Puddings: ice cream (not creamy Cornish varieties), pancakes made with skimmed milk, trifle made with fatless sponge and custard made with skimmed milk, served without cream

Soups: any brand

Yogurts: non-diet varieties

Yorkshire pudding: made with skimmed milk and cooked in a non-stick pan

RED

The following items are high in fat and should only be eaten very occasionally by those who do not need to reduce or watch their weight. Those who *are* trying to lose weight should not eat foods from this list during their weight-reducing campaign, and after that, only very rarely. There are low-fat, healthy alternatives to most of these foods!

Avocado pears
Biscuits, pies, pastries and cakes
Butter and margarine all brands including those low in cholesterol
Chocolate, toffees, fudge, butterscotch
Cream, soured cream, gold top milk
Egg products such as Scotch eggs, crêpes, quiches, pancakes, egg custards
Fat or skin from all meats, poultry, etc.
Fried foods of any kind
Gravy made with meat juices and/or granules
Lard, oil (including vegetable and olive oil), **dripping, suet**
Marzipan
Meat products including salami, pâté, black pudding and all fatty meats such as pork pie, goose
Nuts – all except chestnuts
Oil dressings including French dressing and mayonnaise
Olives
Pancakes made with fat
Peanut butter
Salads served in mayonnaise, French dressing or cream
Sauces made with butter, cream or eggs
Snacks cooked in fat such as crisps, maize etc.
Sunflower seeds

STORE CUPBOARD

The following items are useful to keep in stock since they are common ingredients or accompaniments in low-fat recipes.

Arrowroot
Black pepper in a pepper mill
Brown sauce
Canned mushrooms
Canned tomatoes
Chilli powder
Chilli and garlic sauce
Cornflour
Curry powder
Dried low-fat milk
Fresh herbs and spices (any kind)
Garlic granules and fresh garlic
Gravy powder (not granules)
Ground ginger
Horseradish sauce
Lemon juice
Mint sauce
Mixed dried herbs
Mustard (French and English)
Pasta (egg-free)
Reduced-oil salad dressing
Rice
Salt
Stock cubes (beef, chicken, vegetable and fish)
Sultanas
Tomato ketchup
Tomato purée
White wine vinegar
Vinegar
Yeast extract
In the refrigerator:
Diet drinks
Fresh chopped vegetables (such as carrots, celery, cucumber, peppers and tomatoes)

Fresh fruit
Low-fat cottage cheese
Low-fat fromage frais
Low-fat yogurts
Orange juice (unsweetened)
Sparkling mineral water
Tomato juice

UTENSILS YOU WILL NEED

Chopping board and sharp knife
Garlic press
Kitchen weighing scales
Measuring jug
Non-stick frying pan with a lid
Non-stick saucepans, with lids
Spatula and spoons compatible with non-stick
   pans
Tablespoon and teaspoon for measuring

COOKING TIPS

- Cook without fat at all times. Using non-stick utensils enables you to cook perfectly without it. Use the lid on a saucepan or frying pan to encourage more moisture into the food being prepared. The use of a lid will also help ensure the food is cooked throughout.
- The flavour of some recipes will be further enhanced by allowing the dish to stand after cooking and then reheating before serving. Dishes such as kebabs benefit from soaking in the sauce *before* cooking, in order to absorb maximum flavour (i.e. marinating).
- Remove all skin and fat from chicken and meat BEFORE cooking to avoid the flesh soaking up the fat.
- Use low-fat yogurt in place of single cream in recipes, and low-fat fromage frais in place of double cream. However, never overheat these products.

WHAT WE NEED FOR A HEALTHY DIET

Each day we need an adequate supply of fuel in the form of food to supply us with energy, and we need various nutrients so that all our bodily functions WORK properly and constant repairs and renewals are carried out.

Foods fall into five basic nutritional categories:
- **Proteins** (meat, fish, eggs and cheese) for growth and repair.
- **Carbohydrates** (bread, pasta, rice, potatoes, cereals) for energy and fibre.
- **Vitamins** (vegetables, fruit, bread, meat, fish) for protection against disease and maintenance of various bodily functions.
- **Minerals** (such as iron in liver and calcium in milk) are also essential: e.g. iron for our blood supply, and calcium for sound bones and teeth.
- **Fats** for energy.

We can obtain all the nutrients we need from the first four categories, and all the energy we need from our carbohydrate foods, which means that as a specific category fat may be dropped. This is not to say that we do not need any fat – we do, but only a small amount, and, as fat is found in most foods except vegetables, there is no danger of the body becoming deficient providing a varied and nutritious diet is eaten. In particular, some fatty fishes such as mackerel, tuna and salmon are particularly nutritious and are recommended. However, those trying to reduce their weight should eat them in moderation.

It is important that we don't get too confused or over-anxious about the nutrients we eat. In a country where food is plentiful and varied we are unlikely to be malnourished. However, a simple guide to the ideal content of our daily diet is this:

DAILY NUTRITIONAL REQUIREMENTS

Each day try to incorporate into your diet the following minimum quantities:

- 6 oz (150g) protein food (fish, poultry, meat, cottage cheese, baked beans)
- 12 oz (300g) vegetables (including salad)
- 12 oz (300g) fresh fruit (including fruit juice)
- 6 oz (150g) carbohydrate (bread, cereals, potatoes, rice, pasta)
- ½ pint (10 fl oz/250ml) skimmed or semi-skimmed milk
- 5 oz (125g) low-fat yogurt or an additional ¼ pint (5 fl oz/125ml) skimmed or semi-skimmed milk

Restrict the consumption of eggs to two per week and red meat preferably to two helpings per week. Vegetarians should also consult pages 76-79 for additional advice on basic nutrition.

Bearing all this in mind, from now on try to make the following adjustments to your eating and shopping habits. By doing so you can drastically reduce your calorie intake without actually eating less food:

- Eat three meals a day.
- Stop cooking with fat (see *Cooking Tips*).
- Stop using butter or margarine on bread and instead use sauces or dressings (see page 28).
- Use reduced-oil or low-fat products instead of full-fat varieties, and low-fat alternatives for cooking (see recipes).
- Use skimmed or semi-skimmed milk in place of full-cream milk, except for very young children.
- Don't eat between meals but eat sufficient at mealtimes to satisfy your appetite. Fill up on vegetables with your evening meal so that you eliminate the need to nibble in the evening.

- Use artificial sweeteners in your drinks or reduce by half the amount of sugar you normally take.
- Drink low-calorie drinks in place of high-sugar ones.
- Restrict alcohol intake to 2 drinks per day for men and to 1 per day for women, with 3 additional drinks per week if required for social occasions.
- Use wholemeal products in place of refined ones (for example, bread, rice).

Follow these ten simple rules and you are on the way to a healthier and more beautiful body.

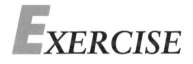

EXERCISE

As part of your preparation for your campaign towards a leaner, fitter and healthier body, not only is it practical to work *gradually* towards commencing your diet, it is also wise to prepare yourself for increased physical activity.

Muscles that have not been exercised for years will prove very painful if overworked when you first start to exercise them again. Such discomfort can quickly discourage any further attempts on the basis that it's too late! We can talk ourselves into believing that the damage and abuse we have caused ourselves over the years is irretrievable. Of course, this is definitely not true. No matter how unfit or unused to physical activity we are, we can change our fitness level surprisingly swiftly if we exercise regularly. Everyone should start slowly and gradually build up their level of activity. Perhaps the most crucial factor is finding a form of exercise you actually enjoy. Exercising to music is my particular favourite and I also work out in our gym twice a week (see pages 185-188). Mike, my husband, plays squash twice a week and works out in the gym whenever he has time. Dawn, my daughter, attends my weekly exercise class and swims twice a week. Exercising shouldn't be a chore but instead should become part of our normal lifestyle. The benefits of regular exercise are obvious: improved fitness, a healthier heart, a toned, more attractive body shape and a higher metabolic rate. Add to this the fact that exercise burns up extra calories . . . so what are we waiting for?

As soon as you have read this chapter, think carefully about how you can increase your physical activity over the next week. Make a list of the exercises you plan to take. Tick each one off as you do it. Here are some suggestions:

- Going for a 20-minute brisk walk
- Swimming for 15 minutes
- Walking up and down stairs 20 times
- Marching on the spot for 5 minutes
- Cycling – outdoors, for 2 miles
- Cycling – indoors, for 3 minutes
- Walking slowly for 1 hour
- Digging the garden for 15 minutes

Aim to do *something* physical each day. Exercise should be energetic enough to make you puff but not cause you to be so out of breath that you cannot talk normally. Keep a record of your activity and the duration, repetitions and intensity. Make a note of how you felt afterwards. If you repeat the same activity on a subsequent day, aim to increase the intensity or duration.

Below is a suggested record sheet. If you can't exercise every day, try to do something on at least 3 days of the week.

RECORDING YOUR PROGRESS

Lastly, it is essential that you keep a record of your weight and inch (centimetre) loss progress. Overleaf you will find a guide to taking your measurements and a Weight and Inch (Centimetre) Loss Record Chart. Learn exactly where to measure yourself, and have a weighing and measuring session every week, at the same time of day. Ideally, enlist the help of your partner, children or a close friend. Hopefully they will provide encouragement when they witness the reality of your progress. At the end of the first month complete the Monthly Weight and Inch (Centimetre) Loss Record Chart and note the progress achieved. If you decide to continue on the Whole Body Programme keep adding the details of your progress.

I would also strongly recommend that you take a 'before' photograph of yourself. Wear something really unflattering and ask your partner or a close friend to take the photograph. When you

DAY	ACTIVITY	DURATION	DISTANCE	COMMENTS
Monday	Brisk walking	30 minutes	To Thorpe crossroads	Felt great
Tuesday	Marching on spot	3 minutes	200 steps	Puffed out
Wednesday	Slow walk	40 minutes	Round the block	Great!
Thursday	Gardening	2 hours	Weeding and digging	Back ached!
Friday	Swimming	15 minutes	10 lengths	Felt fitter
Saturday	Brisk walking	40 minutes	Walked to Thorpe village and back	Felt great
Sunday	Rest day!	—	—	—

receive the print back, no matter how dreadful you think you look, save it for the wonderful day when you will show it with great pride. That day you will be able to look at yourself in the mirror and say 'Don't I look better!'

Your instant reaction may well be 'You have got to be joking! I wouldn't be seen dead in a photograph the way I look now!' but please believe me that when you have lost your excess weight, that photograph will be your prize possession and a reminder never to allow yourself to return to that size.

HOW TO MEASURE YOURSELF

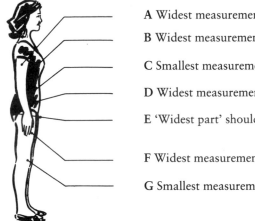

A Widest measurement around the upper arm

B Widest measurement around the bust

C Smallest measurement around the waist

D Widest measurement around the hips

E 'Widest part' should be the largest measurement in this area

F Widest measurement around the thighs

G Smallest measurement above the knees

MONTHLY WEIGHT AND INCH (CENTIMETRE) LOSS RECORD CHART

DATE											
WEIGHT											
WEIGHT LOST THIS MONTH											
INS (CMS) LOST THIS MONTH											
TOTAL WEIGHT LOST TO DATE											
TOTAL INS (CMS) LOST TO DATE											
COMMENTS											

WEIGHT AND INCH (CENTIMETRE) LOSS RECORD CHART

DATE																
WEIGHT																
TOTAL WEIGHT LOST TO DATE																
BUST																
WAIST																
HIPS																
WIDEST PART																
L. THIGH																
R. THIGH																
L. KNEE																
R. KNEE																
L. ARM																
R. ARM																
TOTAL INS (CMS) LOST THIS WEEK																
TOTAL TO DATE																
TOTAL LOSS																

BEFORE PHOTOGRAPH

AFTER PHOTOGRAPH

Date of photograph: _____   Date of photograph: _____
My weight is: _____   My weight is: _____

Date of commencement of diet: _____
Commencing weight: _____
1st Goal Weight: _____stones_____lbs Date achieved_____
2nd Goal Weight: _____stones_____lbs Date achieved_____
3rd Goal Weight: _____stones_____lbs Date achieved_____

Ultimate Goal: _____stones_____lbs Date achieved_____

My reasons for losing weight are:
1. _____
2. _____
3. _____
4. _____
Dates of forthcoming special events:
Date: _____   Event: _____
Date: _____   Event: _____
Date: _____   Event: _____

THE WHOLE BODY PROGRAMME

This 28-Day Whole Body Programme is designed to maximise your reduction of unwanted weight and inches at the same time as increasing your level of energy and fitness.

THE DIET

For each meal in the 28-day diet plan there is a choice of Regular (R), Budget (B) and Vegetarian (V) menus. For starters and desserts to accompany the dinner menus, please see pages 30–31.

Meals may be selected from any of the above categories and may be interchanged from one day to another to suit not only individual tastes but also time and food availability.

The Daily Nutritional Requirements (see page 22) should, however, be observed whenever possible but, providing a varied diet is eaten, malnutrition (bad nutrition) is unlikely to occur.

I would, however, suggest that dieters take one multivitamin tablet each day to make doubly sure they are getting all the vitamins they need.

REMEMBER . . .

- *Do* eat your three meals a day.
- *Do* stick to the menus included in the 28-day plan.
- *Do* try to undertake some form of exercise every day.
- *Do not* eat in between meals.

DIET NOTES

- **Bread**: Whenever possible bread should be wholemeal. For guidance, 1 slice of regular bread from a large thin-sliced loaf weighs 1 oz (25g). A slice from a large medium-sliced loaf weighs 1½ oz (37.5g). Unless otherwise specified in the diet menus, 1 slice equals 1 oz (25g). The term 'light' bread means low-calorie brands such as Nimble or Slimcea.
- **Cottage cheese**: Always select low-fat brands. Flavoured varieties are acceptable but check the nutritional panel for fat content. Avoid cottage cheese mixed with cheddar. Also watch out for brands with cream added!
- **Fruit**: 1 piece of fresh fruit means 1 apple or 1 banana or 4 oz (100g) any fruit such as grapes, strawberries or pineapple.
- **Milk**: For adults milk should be skimmed or semi-skimmed milk – 'Silver top' milk is acceptable providing the cream is removed.

- **Sweeteners**: Low-calorie artificial sweeteners should be used whenever possible in place of sugar.
- **Yogurt**: All yogurts should be low-fat, low-calorie varieties. Check the nutrition details on the side of the carton to make certain of choosing the right one. However, as it is difficult to find low-fat, low-calorie plain yogurt, try to select brands that do not have any added cream.

DAILY ALLOWANCE

- ½ pint (10 fl oz/250ml) skimmed or semi-skimmed milk.
- 5 fl oz (125ml) unsweetened orange or grapefruit juice or 1 whole orange or grapefruit.
- Alcohol: Men may have 2 drinks per day plus 3 bonus drinks per week. Women may have 1 drink per day plus 3 bonus drinks per week. See below for more details.
- For those who do not drink alcohol, additional fruit juices may be consumed daily. See below for more details.

DRINKS

Tea and coffee may be drunk freely if drunk black, or may be drunk white providing the skimmed or semi-skimmed milk allowance is not exceeded. Use artificial sweetener in place of sugar whenever possible, although a small amount of sugar is permissible.

Men may drink 2 alcoholic drinks per day and women 1 drink per day, plus 3 bonus drinks each week. 'One drink' means a single measure of spirit or one glass of wine, or a small glass of sherry or ½ pint (10 fl oz/250ml) of beer or lager. Slimline mixers should always be used and diet drinks may be drunk freely. If you do not drink alcohol, you are allowed 2 (10 fl oz/250ml) addi-

tional fruit juices, e.g. orange, grapefruit or apple juice. You may drink as much water as you like.

SAUCES AND DRESSINGS

The following sauces may be consumed freely:
- Brown sauce
- Mint sauce
- Soy sauce
- Tomato ketchup
- Worcestershire sauce
- Lemon juice
- Vinegar
- Citrus Dressing (see recipe, page 146)
- Oil-free vinaigrette
- Mustard
- Yeast extract

The following may be used in moderation:
- Barbecue Sauce (see recipe, page 109)
- Horseradish sauce (1 teaspoon allowed)
- Pickle sauces
- Sauces (e.g. parsley sauce, white sauce, etc.)
- Gravy (which must be made with powder, not granules, unless a low-fat variety)
- Reduced-oil salad dressing (always use low-fat brands)
- Yogurt Dressing (see recipe, page 146)

BETWEEN-MEAL SNACKS

The following may be consumed in moderation, if you feel peckish between meals:
- Carrots
- Celery
- Cucumber
- Lettuce
- Mushrooms
- Onions
- Peppers

THE FORBIDDEN LIST

These foods are strictly forbidden whilst following the diet unless otherwise stated (e.g. some exceptions are made for vegetarians):

- All butters, margarines low in cholesterol, low-fat spreads or any similar products
- Cream, soured cream, 'Gold top' milk
- Lard, oil (including vegetable/olive, etc.), dripping, suet
- Oil dressings, including French, mayonnaise, salad dressings
- Fat or skin from all meats, poultry, etc.
- Fried foods of any kind
- Biscuits, crispbreads (*except* Rye crispbreads), pies, pastries or cakes
- Chocolate, toffees, fudge, butterscotch
- Lemon curd, peanut butter
- All cheese (*except* low-fat cottage cheese), fromage frais or Quark
- Egg yolk (the whites may be eaten freely), except where included in the diet
- Egg products, e.g. Scotch eggs, crêpes, quiche, pancakes, custards
- Fatty fish including kippers, rollmop herrings, eels, herrings, sardines, bloaters, sprats and whitebait
- Meat products including sausages, salami, pâté, black pudding and all fatty meats including pork pie, goose, beef burgers
- All nuts, (*except* chestnuts) unless otherwise stated in the diet
- Sunflower seeds
- Salads served in mayonnaise, French dressing or cream

THE QUICK AND EASY BASIC DIET

For those who want to lose weight but don't have the time or inclination to prepare special recipes, the following guidelines will offer quick and easy alternatives.

BREAKFASTS

- 1 oz (25g) cereal plus 5 fl oz (125ml) milk in addition to your allowance

OR

- 1½ oz (37.5g) toast spread with 2 teaspoons marmalade

OR

- 4 pieces any fresh fruit

LUNCHES

- 1 jacket potato (any size) topped with either 8 oz (200g) baked beans or 3 oz (75g) cottage cheese

OR

- 4 slices light bread spread with ketchup, low-oil dressing or pickle and made into sandwiches with salad and any of the following:

2 oz (50g) chicken, turkey or lean ham

3 oz (75g) tuna in brine

3 oz (75g) cottage cheese

OR

- ½ pint (250ml) home-made soup plus 2 slices bread

OR

- 5 pieces any fresh fruit

OR

- 1 slimmer's cup-a-soup, 2 pieces fresh fruit and 2 × 5 oz (2 × 125g) diet yogurts

DINNERS

Select one of the following and serve with unlimited vegetables (including potatoes):

- 8 oz (200g) white fish
- 6 oz (150g) chicken, turkey or duck without skin and weighed without bone

- 4 oz (100g) very lean red meat
- 4 oz (100g) lean pork

Select one starter and one dessert from the lists provided below.

STARTERS – LIST A

To accompany any dinner main course and any dessert from Desserts Lists A or B

- Chicken and Mushroom Soup (see recipe, page 100)
- Chicken Soup (see recipe, page 100)
- Crudités (see recipe, page 97) with Garlic or Mint Yogurt Dip (see recipe, page 97)
- ½ a fresh grapefruit
- ½ pint (10 fl oz/250ml) consommé or any clear soup
- Melon with Ginger (see recipe, page 98)
- Melon and Prawn Salad (see recipe, page 98)
- Minty Melon and Yogurt Salad (see recipe, page 98)
- Spicy Mushrooms (see recipe, page 99)
- Wedge of melon

STARTERS – LIST B

To accompany any dinner main course and any dessert from Desserts List A

- Chestnut Pâté (see recipe, page 80)
- Chilled Green Pea Soup (see recipe, page 101)
- Crunchy Vegetable Dip (see recipe, page 98)
- Duck Soup (see recipe, page 101)
- Minestrone Soup (see recipe, page 102)
- Melon with Strawberries (see recipe, page 98)
- Ratatouille (see recipe, page 135)
- Smoked Mackerel Pâté (see recipe, page 97)
- Smoked Mackerel Pâté with salad (see recipe, page 97)
- Smoked trout, served with Cucumber and Strawberry Salad (see recipe, page 133)
- Tuna Pâté with Crudités (see recipe, page 99)
- Waldorf Salad (see recipe, page 99)

DESSERTS – LIST A

To accompany any dinner main course and any starter from Starters Lists A or B

- ½ a melon
- 1 diet yogurt
- 1 diet fromage frais
- 1 piece any fruit
- 2 oz (50g) frozen yogurt
- 4 oz (100g) strawberries or raspberries
- 5 oz (125g) jelly
- Red Fruit Salad (see recipe, page 143)
- Tropical Fruit Salad (see recipe, page 170)

DESSERTS – LIST B

To accompany any dinner main course and any starter from Starters List A

- ½-inch (1.25cm) slice Banana and Sultana Cake (see recipe, page 136)
- ½-inch (1.25cm) slice Kim's Cake (see recipe, page 138)
- 1 oz (25g) ice cream (non-Cornish variety) with 4 oz (100g) fresh fruit
- Apricot and Banana Fool (see recipe, page 136)
- Cheese and Apricot Pears (see recipe, page 90)
- Fruit Brûlée (see recipe, page 136)
- Ginger Sorbet (see recipe, page 137) with melon
- Gooseberry Fool (see recipe, page 137)
- Hot Cherries (see recipe, page 137)

- Low-fat Rice Pudding (see recipe, page 138)
- Mango and Strawberry Bombe (see recipe, page 138)
- Melon Sundae (see recipe, page 140)
- Meringue Basket filled with fresh fruit and topped with 2 oz (50g) diet yogurt
- 2 Meringue Biscuits (see recipe, page 142) with 8 oz (200g) strawberries, topped with 2 oz (50g) diet yogurt
- Oranges Grand Marnier and Yogurt Sauce (see recipe, page 140)
- Peach Brûlée (see recipe, page 140)
- Pears in Meringue (see recipe, page 141)
- Pears in Red Wine (see recipe, page 141)
- Pineapple, Peach and Strawberry Dessert (see recipe, page 141)
- Raspberry Fluff (see recipe, page 141)
- Raspberry Mousse (see recipe, page 142)
- Raspberry Yogurt Delight (see recipe, page 142)
- Strawberry Sorbet (see recipe, page 143)
- Summer Pudding (see recipe, page 143)
- Summer Surprise (see recipe, page 144)

THE EXERCISE PROGRAMME

WHY EXERCISE?

Exercise offers many benefits to everyone. Not only does it provide numerous benefits to our general health, it is particularly effective for those who wish to reduce their size and who are on weight-reducing diets. The following points are especially relevant.

- Exercise helps to burn up valuable extra calories, thus increasing the *speed* of weight and inch (centimetre) loss.
- Aerobic exercise actually works as a fat *burner*. To achieve this we need to work out for 20 minutes, 3 times a week, at a sufficiently energetic level to cause our heart to beat significantly faster than normal.
- Exercise works various groups of muscles, increasing their strength and endurance and helping us to cope more easily with the demands of everyday life such as lifting, working, playing sport and so on.
- 'Worked' muscles become 'toned' muscles and give us a greatly improved body shape.
- Exercise increases the flow of oxygen to the skin and so encourages improved skin tone, which is particularly important when you are losing weight. Sagging skin resulting from weight loss can be prevented by exercise.

EXERCISE FOR OPTIMUM EFFECT

There are five elements contributing to physical fitness. These are stamina, muscular endurance, strength, flexibility and motor fitness.

Stamina
This is built up through sustained aerobic exer-

cise when the body is working hard enough to achieve a heart rate of between 60 per cent and 85 per cent of its maximum. Our maximum heart rate per minute can be calculated by deducting our age from 220.

Muscular endurance

This is developed by training a group of muscles to overcome resistance over a period of time. The source of the resistance can be gravity, our own body weight, or light external weights. To increase muscular endurance as we become fitter we increase the number of repetitions of each exercise.

Strength

Exercises to develop strength can incorporate the use of external weights or we can use our own body weight and gravity to give the necessary resistance. To become *stronger*, we need to increase the resistance and *not* the number of repetitions.

Flexibility

Developing flexibility or suppleness involves the lengthening of muscles by using a wider range of movements, particularly stretching exercises. As we become more supple we are able to stretch the muscles further.

Motor fitness

The relationship between the brain and the muscle action defines our level of motor fitness as it relates to co-ordination, balance and the reaction time taken in the performance of different movements.

The weekly exercise plans in this Whole Body Programme have been created to incorporate all these various elements towards total physical fitness.

THE WORKOUT

The weekly workout plans in this Whole Body Programme have been specially designed on the basis of the most up-to-date opinions of experts in the field of exercise. The aim of these exercise plans is to achieve the optimum benefits for our body not only in terms of mobility, fitness and wellbeing, but also, and perhaps more importantly to some, to improve our physical appearance. This is truly a *whole body* programme.

There are four workout plans, one for each week of the diet. Each week's plan is progressive and allows you to increase your fitness in a controlled way. For maximum benefit try to exercise every day, gradually increasing the intensity and repetitions of the exercises as described in the instructions. If daily practice is impractical, aim to work out at least 3 times a week.

These exercises are designed to cater for various levels of physical fitness. We should work out only within our individual capability and, as we are not training to become Olympic athletes, we should NEVER push ourselves too far. Listen to the natural warning signals given by the body and never exercise beyond your own limits. Remember, our aim is an improved body, not a world record! Each of the four weekly workouts given here includes a warm-up section, an aerobic section, muscular strength and endurance exercises, stretches and remobilising movements. These basic components will give you the following physical benefits:

THE WARM-UP

Warming up our body with gentle exercises prepares the body and mind for exercise, enabling us to maximise our performance both physically and mentally. Warming-up exercises prepare the heart and lungs for the additional work they will have to do; help to prevent soreness and injury in the major muscle groups; and rehearse the movements of the exercises that will follow, thus enhancing our performance. Exercises performed correctly are obviously more effective.

There are three elements of a warm-up:

- **1 Mobilising.** When we take our joints gently through a range of movements the body prepares them for action in various ways, including secreting synovial fluid which allows the joint actions to be smoother, easier and safer.
- **2 Pulse raising.** By practising a few exercises that use the large muscle groups we increase our heart rate and prepare our cardiovascular system for exercise.
- **3 Preparatory stretches.** We need to stretch our muscles to reduce the chance of injury. Muscles are like elastic and become more pliable when warm. Warming and stretching them prevents injury and improves performance.

AEROBIC SECTION

Aerobic exercise strengthens our heart and also burns body fat. It improves the capacity and efficiency of the cardiorespiratory system so that it delivers more oxygen to the working muscles. It improves muscular endurance, lowers our blood fat levels and helps to lower blood pressure. There are also various other benefits in the reduction of risk factors associated with coronary heart disease.

The energy source of aerobic exercise is oxygen. We breathe more heavily during aerobic exercise because the body demands a greater supply of oxygen. Providing the oxygen supply is maintained, aerobic exercise can be continued for a long time (as in the case of a marathon runner). Aerobic exercise involves the larger muscle groups (those of the arms and legs) and can be high-impact or low-impact, high-intensity or low-intensity. High-impact aerobic exercises involve both feet leaving the ground (e.g. jumping, jogging or skipping) whereas low-impact exercise is when one foot always remains on the floor (e.g. a walking jog, knee raises or marching). The intensity level is determined by the size and speed of a movement. Someone who finds it difficult to do high-impact aerobics can still work out very energetically if large and high arm movements are included.

The aerobic exercises recommended here can be adapted to your individual capability. If you do not wish to perform high-impact movements, keep the exercises low-impact by eliminating the skip, jump or jogging element. Instead, just step or walk.

MUSCULAR STRENGTH AND ENDURANCE EXERCISES

Muscular strength and endurance exercises help our muscles to support our skeleton and maintain our posture and shape. It is these exercises that will particularly improve our figure. However, not only could they be harmful but they will not be as effective if we do not warm up properly, so do not do them in isolation.

STRENGTH exercises will obviously make our muscles stronger, whilst ENDURANCE exercises enable the muscles to participate in continuous activity for longer. Both strength and endurance exercises improve our muscle tone.

To progress with STRENGTH exercises we need to increase the resistance as we get fitter but to do only a few repetitions. To progress in ENDURANCE exercises we should increase the number of repetitions but keep the resistance low.

STRETCHING

After we have worked our muscles hard through the aerobic and muscular strength and endurance exercises we need to stretch them out again to return them to their normal state. It is also important to encourage our muscles to be used in an extended form as well as in a contraction. Otherwise bad posture could result, with long-term detrimental effects to our body shape.

Some stretches should be held in the extreme position for a minimum of 6 to 8 seconds; others can be held for longer and even progressed still further. This second group are called developmental stretches. Whilst these are beneficial for some muscles, it isn't so for all of them. You will see from the stretches I have included in the 4-week programme which ones belong to this category.

REMOBILISING

After a full workout it is recommended that we remobilise the major joints of our body for two or three minutes. This helps us to rid the body of any waste products created by the exercises and increases our circulation.

If you can remobilise your body to some fun, lively music you will finish your workout feeling on top of the world!

MUSIC AND EXERCISE

There is absolutely no doubt that exercising to music is infinitely more enjoyable than working out in silence. It supplies a regular beat to help us exercise rhythmically. There is also a psychological benefit, as those who exercise to music find they can continue for longer, therefore achieving even greater benefits.

RECORDING YOUR PROGRESS

Record your progress by making a pencil note alongside each exercise recording the number of steps or repetitions you are able to do each time you work out. If you prefer, you could keep a record in a small notebook, logging the week number and the number of the exercise and the number of repetitions or steps. You'll be greatly encouraged when you see how quickly you become fitter.

Be sure to weigh and measure yourself at the beginning of the 4-week programme and, ideally, have a photograph taken of you in your 'before' state. You don't have to show it to anyone, but when you have achieved your new body shape you'll be proud to show it.

TEN ESSENTIAL TIPS FOR EXERCISING

• **1** Always check with your doctor before starting this or any other kind of exercise and diet programme. If during the exercises you feel any pain or discomfort, stop immediately. If you feel one particular exercise doesn't suit you because it is uncomfortable to do, leave it out.

• **2** Movements should always be rhythmic, controlled and slow, never jerky or hurried. To do so eliminates the benefits.

• **3** ALWAYS warm up before any form of exercise.

• **4** Never overwork or overstretch your body. Look for warning signals such as feeling faint, pain, nausea and so on.

• **5** Relate the level of your workout to your environment (e.g. type of flooring, fresh air, heat, etc.) and your own physical condition. If you haven't exercised for 30 years, take it very slowly at the start and increase your activity as you become fitter.

• **6** Always wear suitable clothing for exercise. Correct footwear is particularly important, especially for aerobic exercise.

• **7** If you become fit enough to do many repetitions of some of the exercises included in this programme, beware of possible overuse of some of your joints. To remedy this, go on to the next exercise that uses different muscles and joints, then return to the original exercise. Vary the high-impact and low-impact aerobic exercises in the same way.

• **8** You should be able to feel the muscle that is 'working' in the strength and endurance exercises. If you can't, check that you are doing the exercise correctly by carefully rereading the instructions. Do the same with the stretching exercises. If you can't feel the muscle being stretched, double check your position with that in the picture.

• **9** Plan a time to do your exercises each day and try to stick to it. Be disciplined about your workout. This is your opportunity to have a great new body in just 4 weeks. Work out with a friend or partner for greater enjoyment. The exercises are suitable for men and women.

• **10** Never exercise immediately after a meal. Wait at least 1 to 1½ hours.

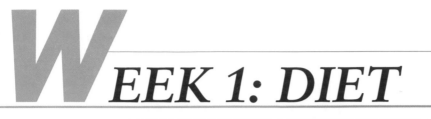

WEEK 1: DIET

It is important that you weigh and measure yourself in the morning on the day you begin this Whole Body Programme. Do this before you eat or drink anything to get your most accurate reading, then enter the details on the Weight and Inch (Centimetre) Loss Record Chart on page 25.

DAY 1

BREAKFASTS
(R) 1 rasher bacon, grilled, plus 3 grilled tomatoes and 1 slice toast
(B) 1 oz (25g) any cereal plus ¼ pint (5 fl oz/125ml) milk in addition to allowance, 1 teaspoon sugar
(V) 4 pieces any fresh fruit

LUNCHES
(R) Cucumber Boats with Tuna (see recipe, page 94), served with salad
(B) Mixed Vegetable Soup (see recipe, page 102) plus 1 slice bread or toast
(V) 2 slices bread spread with Marmite and topped with 4 oz (100g) cottage cheese and grated carrot

DINNERS
(R) Prawn Pilaff (see recipe, page 123)
(B) Chicken Italienne (see recipe, page 113) – save all bones for soup on Day 3
(V) Vegetable Risotto (see recipe, page 132)

DAY 2

BREAKFASTS
(R) 1 wholemeal bread roll (approx. 2 oz/50g) spread with mustard and 1 oz (25g) lean ham
(B) 1 slice (1½ oz/37.5g) toast plus 2 teaspoons marmalade
(V) 8 oz (200g) natural yogurt mixed with ¼ oz (6.5g) oats (dry porridge) and ½ oz (12.5g) sultanas and 1 teaspoon honey

LUNCHES
(R) 5 pieces any fresh fruit
(B) 1 slice toast topped with 8 oz (200g) baked beans plus 1 piece fresh fruit
(V) 8 oz Creamy Vegetable Soup (see recipe, page 101) plus 2 Ryvitas spread with Marmite

DINNERS
(R) Spicy Pork Volcano (see recipe, page 108), served with rice mixed with beansprouts
(B) Chicken Pilaff (see recipe, page 113)
(V) Stir-fried Vegetables with Ginger and Sesame Marinade (see recipe, page 85)

DAY 3

BREAKFASTS
(R) 1 boiled egg plus 1 slice toast
(B) 1 wholemeal bread roll (approx. 2 oz/50g) spread with 2 teaspoons preserve (jam, honey or marmalade)
(V) 1 slice toast plus 5 oz (125g) baked beans

LUNCHES
(R) 1 slimmer's cup-a-soup plus 2 Ryvitas spread with Marmite and topped with 2 oz (50g) cottage cheese, plus 1 piece fresh fruit and 5 oz (125g) diet yogurt
(B) ½ pint (10 fl oz/250ml) Chicken Soup (see recipe, page 100) plus 2 slices toast
(V) 4 pieces any fresh fruit plus 5 oz (125g) plain yogurt

DINNERS
(R) Chicken and Mushroom Supreme (see recipe, page 110), served with unlimited vegetables
(B) Barbecued Fish Kebabs (see recipe, page 119), served with boiled rice cooked in water flavoured with fish stock cube
(V) Cauliflower and Courgette Bake (see recipe, page 127)

DAY 4

BREAKFASTS

(**R**) ¾ oz (20g) any cereal plus 1 sliced banana, served with just under ¼ pint (4 fl oz/ 100ml) milk in addition to allowance. No sugar
(**B**) 1 oz (25g) Porridge (see recipe, page 90)
(**V**) 8 oz (200g) fresh fruit salad plus 5 oz (125g) plain yogurt or a 'petit' fromage frais

LUNCHES

(**R**) Club Sandwich (see recipe, page 92)
(**B**) 2 slices (2 × 1½ oz/ 75g) bread spread with reduced-oil salad dressing and filled with 3 oz (75g) cottage cheese and salad
(**V**)Rice Salad (see recipe, page 96)

DINNERS

(**R**) Cod Parcels (see recipe, page 120), served with unlimited vegetables
(**B**) Stir-fried Chicken and Vegetables (see recipe, page 119), served with boiled rice
(**V**)Tricolour Pasta Risotto (see recipe, page 88)

DAY 5

BREAKFASTS

(**R**) 2 × 5 oz (2 × 125g) diet yogurts placed in a bowl with 1 chopped apple and one sliced banana added
(**B**) 1 slice toast plus 1 poached egg
(**V**) 8 oz (200g) natural yogurt mixed with 10 sultanas and 1 teaspoon honey

LUNCHES

(**R**) Savoury French Bread Rings (see recipe, page 96)
(**B**) 1 jacket potato (any size) topped with 8 oz (200g) baked beans. NB: while baking the jacket potato in the oven, cook a Banana and Sultana Cake (see recipe, page 136)
(**V**) 4 slices light bread spread with reduced-oil salad dressing, filled with sliced beetroot, tomatoes and 1 egg, hard-boiled

DINNERS

(**R**) Barbecued Beef Kebabs (see recipe for Barbecued Kebabs, page 102), served with 2 oz (50g) boiled rice and 4 oz (100g) beansprouts
(**B**) Chicken Pilaff (see recipe, page 113)
(**V**) Bean and Vegetable Bake (see recipe, page 126)

DAY 6

BREAKFASTS

(**R**) ½ melon topped with 4 oz (100g) seedless grapes and a melon-flavoured diet yogurt
(**B**) 2 slices toast spread with Marmite
(**V**) 1 slice (1½ oz/37.5g) toast topped with 16 oz (400g) tinned tomatoes and 5 oz (125g) tinned mushrooms

LUNCHES

(**R**) Salad Surprise (see recipe, page 96)
(**B**) 2 pieces fresh fruit plus 2 × ½ in (1.25cm) slices Banana and Sultana Cake (see recipe, page 136)
(**V**) ½ pint (10 fl oz/250ml) Creamy Vegetable Soup (see recipe, page 101) and 1 slice toast, plus 1 piece fresh fruit and 5 oz (125g) natural yogurt

DINNERS

(**R**) Trout with Apples (see recipe, page 124), served with unlimited vegetables
(**B**) Fish Cakes (see recipe, page 121), served with unlimited vegetables
(**V**) Duo of Courgettes and Flageolets en Salade (see recipe, page 82)

DAY 7

BREAKFASTS

(**R**) 8 oz (200g) fresh fruit salad mixed with 6 oz (150g) natural yogurt or 1 diet yogurt, any flavour
(**B**) 2 Weetabix plus ¼ pint (5 fl oz/125ml) milk in addition to allowance, plus 2 teaspoons sugar
(**V**) ½ melon chopped and mixed with 1 oz (25g) sultanas, 3 chopped walnuts and 5 oz (125g) natural yogurt

LUNCHES

(**R**) Smoked Mackerel Pâté (see recipe, page 97), served with 1 slice toast and salad
(**B**) 4 Ryvitas spread with Marmite and topped with 1 egg, hard-boiled and sliced
(**V**) 2 slices toast topped with 8 oz (200g) baked beans and 4 oz (100g) tinned tomatoes boiled down to a creamy consistency

DINNERS

(**R**) Chicken à l'Orange (see recipe, page 109), served with unlimited vegetables
(**B**) Chicken Curry (see recipe, page 112)
(**V**) Vegetable Kebabs (see recipe, page 131), served with boiled brown rice and sweetcorn

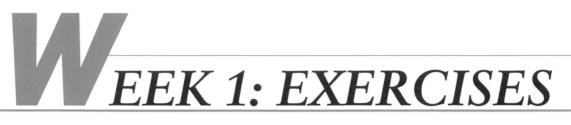

WEEK 1: EXERCISES

WARM-UP I: MOBILISER

Before you start your first week of exercises make sure you have read and understood the notes and instructions at the beginning of this chapter. Ideally, put aside a set time each day to practise. Start off gently on the first day and try to do as many of the exercises as you can, gradually increasing the number of repetitions each day as you become fitter.

Enjoy yourself!

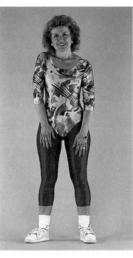

1 Shoulder raises Standing with your feet slightly apart and your knees slightly bent, raise and lower one shoulder 8 times. Repeat with the other shoulder.

2 Shoulder rotation backwards Rotate one shoulder backwards 8 times then repeat with the other shoulder.

3 Shoulder rotation forwards Rotate one shoulder forwards 8 times then repeat with the other shoulder.

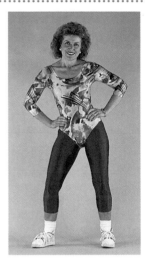

4 Pelvic rotation With hands on hips, rotate your hips 4 times in a clockwise direction and then 4 times in an anti-clockwise direction. Repeat in both directions for 4 rotations each way.

WARM-UP II: PULSE RAISER

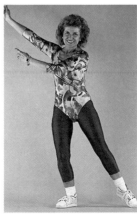

7 Swing and point Swing arms from side to side, shifting your weight on to alternate feet and pointing the foot of the straight leg. Repeat 16 times.

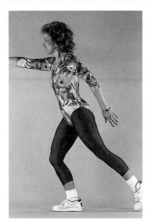

8 Low-impact spotty dog Alternately swing one arm forwards as you step back with the opposite foot. Repeat 16 times (8 on each foot).

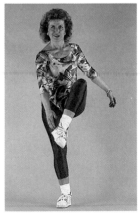

9 Alternate foot raises Raise one foot towards the opposite hand then repeat with the other foot. Repeat 16 times (8 with each foot).

THE WARM-UP

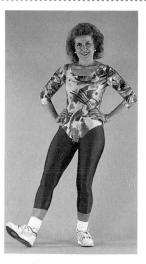 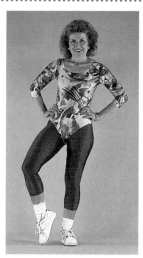 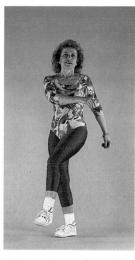

5 Heel and toe tapping
With hands on hips, tap the
heel of one foot and

then the toe. Repeat 8 times
(8 heels and 8 toes) and
then repeat with the other
foot.

6 Arm swinging, knee raises
Swinging your arms gently
from side to side, raise
alternate knees across your
body. Repeat with alternate
legs 16 times (8 raises for
each leg).

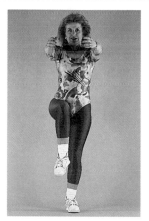

*10 Marching, arms out and
in* Marching on the spot
with large steps, take your
arms out to the sides then
into the centre. Repeat 24
times (12 with each leg).

THE WARM-UP AND AEROBIC WORKOUT

WARM-UP III: PREPARATORY STRETCHES

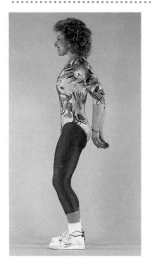 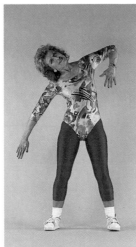 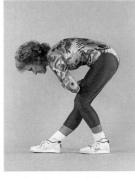 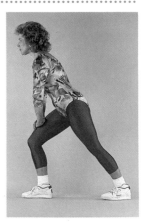

13 *Hamstring stretch*
Standing with one foot behind the other and with your feet hip-width apart, feet pointing straight ahead, keep the front leg straight and bend the back leg, lowering your hips without straining. Place your hands on your thigh (not on your knee) and hold for 6 seconds. Slowly straighten up then proceed to the next exercise.

11 *Chest stretch* Standing with your knees slightly bent and your arms hanging by your sides, draw your shoulders back stretching the muscles across your upper chest. Hold for 6 seconds then relax.

12 *Waist stretch* Standing with your knees slightly bent, slowly curve your spine sideways and hold for 6 seconds. Slowly straighten up then curve your spine over to the other side and hold for 6 seconds. Relax.

14 *Calf stretch* Step back further with the back leg and bend your front knee. Keep feet pointing straight ahead. Ensuring the back leg is straight with heel flat on the floor, bend the front knee over your ankle. do not strain. Hold for 6 seconds. Repeat Exercises 13 and 14 with the other leg.

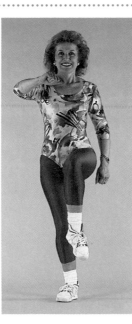 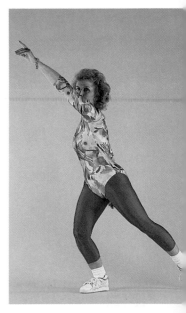

16 *Marching* March on the spot with big steps, swinging your arms in large movements as you march. Continue for as many steps as possible. Record your number of steps and try to increase the number each time you exercise.

AEROBIC WORKOUT

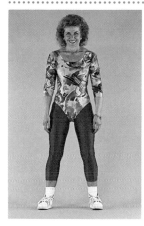

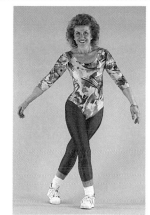

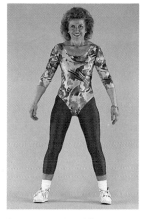

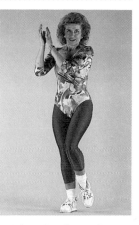

15 *The grapevine* This is a 3-steps-and-a-skip movement. Standing with feet comfortably apart, step out sideways with your right foot.

Then place your left foot behind your right one.

Step out again with your right foot.

Finish with a skip and a clap. Repeat the sequence 4 times in each direction.

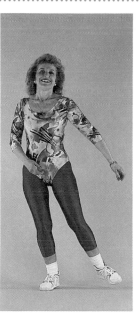

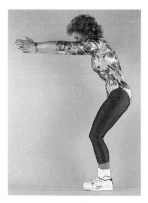

17 *Lungeing* Swing your left arm across and upwards at the same time as stepping out sideways with your left leg. Repeat to the other side with your right arm reaching across and your right leg stepping out sideways. Repeat as many times as possible, increasing the number with each workout. Record your progress.

18 *Sideways jogging* Jog from side to side, allowing your arms to swing with you. Repeat as many times as possible. Record the number of repetitions and try to do more each time you exercise.

The following exercise allows your pulse rate to lower gradually before you progress to the exercises for specific body areas.

19 *Ski down* Pulling your tummy in, raise both arms above your head and gently swing them down by your sides as you bend your knees. Slowly reach up as you straighten again and repeat the exercise 12 times.

MUSCULAR STRENGTH AND ENDURANCE

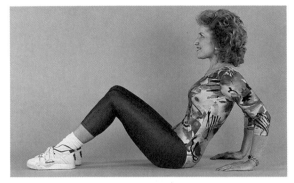

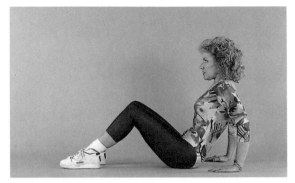

20 *Tricep dip* Sit with your knees bent and feet flat on the floor. Place your hands on the floor behind you, fingers pointing towards your feet. Slowly bend and then straighten the arms, without locking the elbows. Repeat this bending and straightening movement 8 times. Keep your tummy pulled in throughout the exercise.

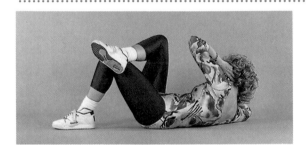

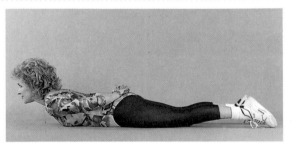

23 *Waist whittler* Bend your knees and place your feet flat on the floor. Raise your right leg and place it in front of the left leg. Place your hands to the sides (not the back) of your head and raise, to the count of 2, your left shoulder towards the right knee. Lower to the count of 2. Repeat 8 times, then slowly change over the position of your legs. Repeat the exercise, raising right shoulder towards left knee.

24 *Back strengthener* Roll over on to your front and place your hands (palms upwards) in the small of your back. Slowly raise your head and shoulders from the floor to the count of 3 then gently lower to the floor. Repeat as many times as you can comfortably. Record the number of repetitions each time you exercise.

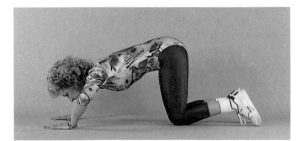

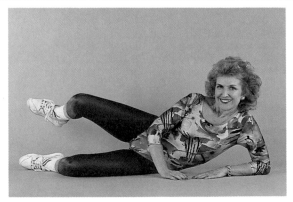

26 *Press-ups* Position yourself as shown, placing your hands wider, but in line with your shoulders. Keeping your back straight, slowly lower your chest towards the floor then raise up again. Do not 'lock' your elbows. Repeat as to ability.

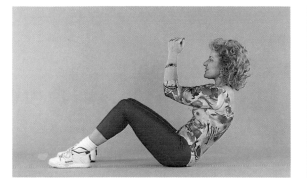

21 Tummy toner Sit with your knees bent and feet flat on the floor. Pulling your tummy in, slowly lean backwards while moving your bent arms in and out to the sides as if playing a concertina. Keep your elbows at shoulder level and work out a rhythm which suits your ability.

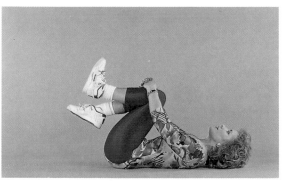

22 Alternate flex and point This exercise strengthens the front of your calves. Lie down on the floor and cuddle your knees. As you do so, flex and point each foot alternately. Repeat 16 times (8 each foot).

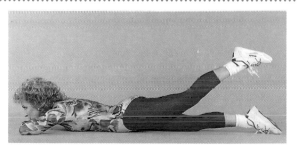

25 Bottom and thigh toner Lying face down on the floor with legs out straight, head on hands, slowly raise one leg, keeping it as straight as possible.

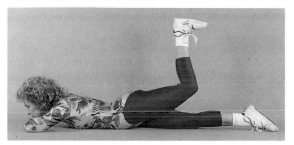

Slowly bend the raised leg (do not point the toe), then straighten it again and slowly lower it to the floor. Repeat with the other leg. Repeat 16 times in all, alternating legs.

27 Outer thigh streamliner Lie on your side, either propping yourself up on your elbow or lying with your arm outstretched above your head. Bend both legs then raise the top leg towards the ceiling. Keep the knees and hips facing forwards at all times, *not* pointing towards the ceiling. Lower your leg slowly. Repeat 8 times, increasing the number of repetitions as you get fitter. Record your repetitions. Proceed to the next exercise, then roll over and repeat Exercises 27 and 28 with the other leg.

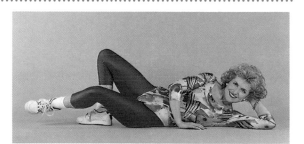

28 Inner thigh streamliner Place the upper leg behind the lower leg with its foot flat on the floor. Slowly raise the lower leg, still bent, as far as possible. Lower it gently. Repeat 8 times to begin with, increasing with practice.

STRETCHES

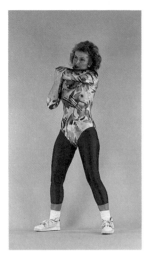

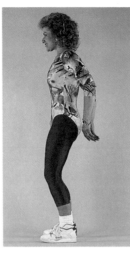

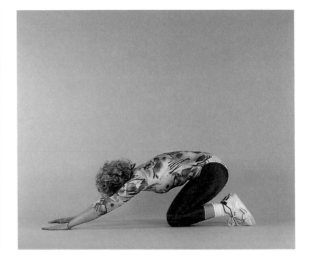

29 Tricep stretch Either standing or sitting, place one arm across your chest. Take hold of it with the opposite hand and stretch it a little further. Hold for 8 seconds. Slowly lower it then change arms.

30 Chest stretch Either standing with your knees slightly bent or sitting on the floor, draw your shoulders back as though trying to get your shoulder blades to touch. Hold for 8 seconds then slowly release.

31 Cat stretch Position yourself on your hands and knees then slowly stretch back like a cat, without sitting on your heels. Hold the stretch for 8 seconds then relax.

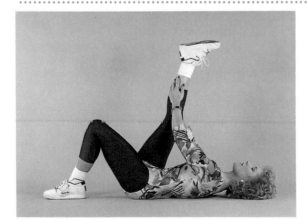

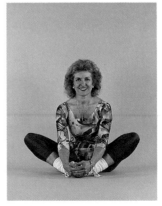

34 Hamstring stretch Start with both knees bent and feet flat on the floor. Bring one bent leg towards your chest, slowly straighten it and hold in the extreme position. If your leg begins to shake, relax it a little, as this is the body's warning system to say you have overstretched it. After 10 seconds you will find the muscle has relaxed and you may be able to stretch it a little further. If so, hold it in the extended position for a further 10 seconds. Slowly bend and lower the leg then repeat with the other leg.

35 Inner thigh stretch Sit up and place the soles of your feet together. Slowly try to lower your knees towards the floor. Hold the position for 10 seconds then try to lower a little further without straining. Hold for a further 10 seconds then relax.

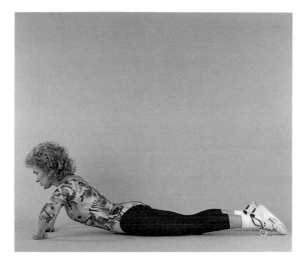

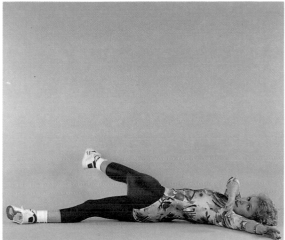

32 Half cobra This exercise stretches your abdominal muscles. Lie on the floor on your tummy and place your hands under your shoulders (fingers pointing inwards). Slowly curl backwards but do not go very far. Do *not* attempt to straighten your arms. Hold for 8 seconds then gradually lower yourself to the floor.

33 Waist and thigh stretch Roll over and lie on your back. Slowly allow your arms to drop to your left side while you bend and raise your left leg and allow it to extend over your body towards your right side. Do not strain and do not attempt to touch the floor with your left foot. Hold for 8 seconds. Slowly bend your leg and bring your arms and leg back to a resting position. Repeat to the other side.

REMOBILISE

Turn back to pages 38-39 and repeat Exercises 1–6. Perform just a few repetitions of each movement to remobilise your joints and leave your body feeling great.

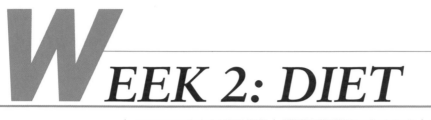

WEEK 2: DIET

You have now completed a week of this Whole Body Programme and, already, you should be feeling slimmer and fitter. Before you commence week two of the programme remember to weigh and measure yourself and enter the details on the Weight and Inch (Centimetre) Loss Record Chart on page 25).

DAY 8

BREAKFASTS
(R) 4 Ryvitas spread with 2 teaspoons pickle, topped with 1½ oz (37.5g) cooked chicken breast or lean ham
(B) ½ oz (12.5g) cereal served with milk from allowance and 1 teaspoon sugar, plus 1 slice toast spread with preserve
(V) 6 oz (150g) plain yogurt mixed with 1 sliced banana and 1 oz (25g) sultanas

LUNCHES
(R) Triple-decker sandwich (3 slices bread spread with oil-free pickle and reduced-oil salad dressing and filled with 1 oz (25g) turkey or chicken roll, plus salad)
(B) 2 slices toast topped with 8 oz (200g) canned spaghetti in tomato sauce
(V) Chilli Salad (see recipe, page 91)

DINNERS
(R) Barbecued Pork Kebabs (see recipe for Barbecued Kebabs, page 102), served with boiled rice and beansprouts
(B) Shepherd's Pie (see recipe, page 107), served with unlimited vegetables
(V) Rice and Almond Pilaff (see recipe, page 81)

DAY 9

BREAKFASTS
(R) Porridge (see recipe, page 90)
(B) 4 Ryvitas spread with 4 teaspoons marmalade
(V) 1½ oz (37.5g) any cereal (inc. muesli) and ¼ pint (5 fl oz/125ml) milk in addition to allowance, plus 1 teaspoon sugar

LUNCHES
(R) 4 slices light bread spread with reduced-oil salad dressing and filled with 2 oz (50g) chopped chicken breast mixed with 2 tablespoons sweetcorn
(B) 2 oz (50g) cooked chicken, plus Coleslaw (see recipe, page 133) and 4 oz (100g) hot or cold cooked potatoes
(V) Sweetcorn and red bean salad (mix the drained contents of a small can of sweetcorn and a small can of red kidney beans together). Serve with a green salad

DINNERS
(R) Savoury Meat Loaf (see recipe, page 107) with unlimited vegetables
(B) 1 Mini Pizza (see recipe, page 106), served with salad
(V) Vegetable Curry (see recipe, page 130), served with boiled rice

DAY 10

BREAKFASTS
(R) ½ fresh grapefruit plus 1 small egg, poached or boiled, served with 1 slice toast spread with Marmite
(B) 2 Weetabix spread with 1 tablespoon preserve and eaten as biscuits
(V) 1 oz (25g) bran cereal, served with ¼ pint (5 fl oz/125ml) milk in addition to allowance and 1 teaspoon sugar

LUNCHES
(R) Curried Chicken and Yogurt Salad (see recipe, page 94)
(B) 4 slices light bread or 2 slices regular bread, made into sandwiches with Coleslaw (see recipe, page 133), lettuce and sliced tomatoes
(V) 4 Ryvitas thinly spread with low-fat soft cheese and topped with salad

DINNERS
(R) Fillet of Beef with Peppercorns (see recipe, page 103), served with unlimited vegetables
(B) Barbecued Chicken Kebabs (see recipe, page 109), served with boiled rice and grilled tomatoes
(V) Fresh Tagliatelle with Blue Cheese Sauce (see recipe, page 81)

DAY 11

BREAKFASTS
(R) 6 oz (150g) tinned grapefruit in natural juice topped with 5 oz (125g) grapefruit yogurt
(B) 1 slice toast spread with 2 teaspoons preserve or Marmite, plus 1 piece fresh fruit
(V) 4 Ryvitas spread with Marmite and topped with 3 oz (75g) cottage cheese

LUNCHES
(R) 4 slices light bread spread with reduced-oil salad dressing, filled with 3 oz (75g) tinned salmon, and cucumber
(B) 1 × 12 oz (300g) can any branded soup (except cream varieties), with 1 wholemeal roll
(V) Jacket potato with 2 oz (50g) sweetcorn mixed with chopped green pepper, 2 oz (50g) cottage cheese and 1 tablespoon reduced-oil salad dressing

DINNERS
(R) Savoury Oven-baked Chicken Legs (see recipe, page 118), served with unlimited vegetables
(B) Spicy Spaghetti Bolognese (see recipe, page 108)
(V) Quick and Low-fat Courgette Lasagne (see recipe, page 84)

DAY 12

BREAKFASTS
(R) 5 prunes in natural juice topped with 5 oz (125g) diet yogurt
(B) 1 oz (25g) any cereal with ¼ pint (5 fl oz/ 125ml) milk in addition to allowance, plus 1 teaspoon sugar
(V) 1 oz (25g) any cereal mixed with 5 oz (125g) natural yogurt and 1 teaspoon honey

LUNCHES
(R) Chicken Liver Salad (see recipe, page 91)
(B) 4 Ryvitas spread with Marmite or reduced-oil salad dressing topped with 2 oz (50g) cottage cheese, plus ½-inch (1.25cm) slice Banana and Sultana Cake (see recipe, page 136)
(V) Kiwifruit Mousse (see recipe, page 95) served with green salad

DINNERS
(R) Prawn Stir-fry (see recipe, page 124), served with boiled rice
(B) Chicken Chop Suey (see recipe, page 112)
(V) Broccoli Gratiné with Cheese and Cannellini Topping (see recipe, page 86)

DAY 13

BREAKFASTS
(R) 4 oz (100g) baked beans and 4 oz (100g) tinned tomatoes, served on 1 slice toast
(B) 1 slice toast spread with Marmite and topped with sliced tomatoes
(V) 4 Ryvitas spread with 1 teaspoon jam or honey mixed with 4 oz (100g) cottage cheese

LUNCHES
(R) 2 slices bread spread with Marie Rose Dressing (see recipe, page 146), filled with 4 oz (100g) peeled prawns and lettuce
(B) 5 Ryvitas spread with reduced-oil dressing, topped with 3 oz (75g) cottage cheese and salad
(V) 8 oz (200g) cold baked beans, served with a large side-salad with 2 teaspoons reduced-oil dressing, plus 5 oz (125g) natural yogurt

DINNERS
(R) Chicken with Orange and Apricots (see recipe, page 114), served with unlimited vegetables
(B) Liver and Onion Casserole (see recipe, page 105), served with unlimited vegetables
(V) Vegetable Pilaff (see recipe, page 131)

DAY 14

BREAKFASTS
(R) Home-made Muesli (see recipe, page 89)
(B) 1 Weetabix plus ½ oz (12.5g) any other cereal, served with ¼ pint (5 fl oz/ 125ml) milk in addition to allowance, and 1 teaspoon sugar
(V) ½ grapefruit plus 3 Ryvitas with 3 teaspoons marmalade

LUNCHES
(R) Jacket potato topped with 1 oz (25g) cooked chicken mixed with 2 oz (50g) natural yogurt, 1 tablespoon reduced-oil salad dressing and 1 teaspoon curry powder
(B) 2 slices toast with 8 oz (200g) baked beans
(V) 8 oz (200g) cottage cheese mixed with 1 pear, 1 apple and 2 sticks celery, chopped, served on a bed of lettuce, with tomatoes and cucumber

DINNERS
(R) Oriental Prawn Salad (see recipe, page 122), served with Minty Melon and Yogurt Salad (see recipe, page 98)
(B) Chicken and Potato Pie (see recipe, page 111), served with unlimited vegetables
(V) Mixed Grain and Fresh Coriander Medley (see recipe, page 85)

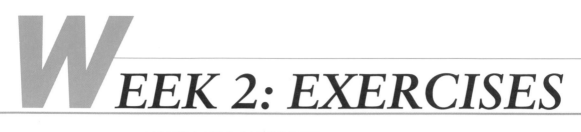

WEEK 2: EXERCISES

I hope you were able to attempt most of the exercises in last week's workout. This week you will find that the exercises have progressed slightly in order to give your muscles a little extra work so that your body will become fitter and more shapely. If at all possible try to do all the exercises in this week's programme every day. Remember, exercise burns extra calories and makes us look and feel better. Have a good week!

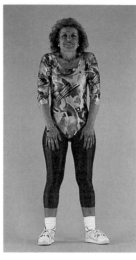

1 Shoulder raises Standing with your feet hip-width apart and your knees slightly bent, raise both shoulders upwards then lower them again. Repeat the movement 8 times and then continue by raising each shoulder alternately for 16 raises (8 for each shoulder).

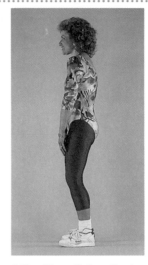

2 Shoulder rolls Standing in the same position as in Exercise 1, roll both shoulders simultaneously in a forwards direction 8 times and then roll them backwards 8 times. Repeat 8 more times forwards and backwards.

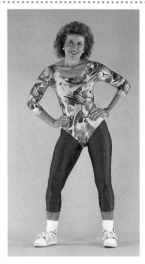

3 Pelvic rotation With your hands on your hips, rotate your hips 4 times in a clockwise direction and then 4 times in an anti-clockwise direction. Repeat this movement with 4 more rotations in each direction.

WARM-UP III: PREPARATORY STRETCHES

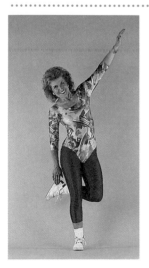

8 Kick and touch Kick your left leg behind the right one and try to touch the foot with your right hand; at the same time allow your left hand to swing upwards. Repeat to the other side. Repeat this sequence 20 times (10 for each leg).

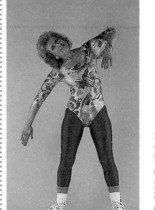

9 Waist stretch Standing with your knees slightly bent, slowly curve your spine sideways and hold the position for 6 seconds. Slowly straighten up then curve over to the other side and hold for 6 seconds. Relax.

THE WARM-UP

WARM-UP II: PULSE RAISER

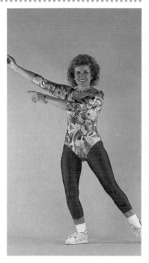

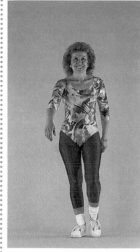

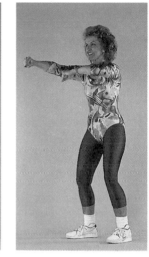

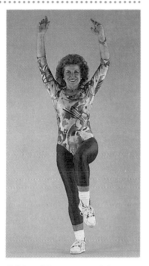

4 *Swing and point* Swinging your arms gently from side to side, move your weight on to alternate feet and point the foot of the straight leg. Repeat 16 times (8 to each side).

5 *Walking jog* Do a walking jog on the spot for 30 steps (15 with each foot). Swing your arms as you step.

6 *Punching* Standing with your feet comfortably apart, knees slightly bent and tummy pulled in, raise your arms to shoulder level and punch forwards with alternate arms. Repeat 20 times (10 for each arm).

7 *Marching, arm raising* Marching on the spot with big leg movements, raise your arms out to the sides and up above your head then down as you place each foot back on the floor. Repeat 20 times (10 for each foot).

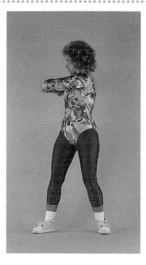

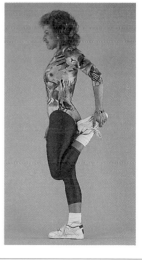

10 *Waist twist* Stand with your feet apart and knees slightly bent. Raise your arms to shoulder level in front and bend your elbows so they point out to the sides. Slowly twist your upper body to one side and hold the position for 6 seconds. Slowly return to the central position then twist to the opposite side and hold for 6 seconds. Slowly return to the centre and relax.

11 *Front thigh stretch* Standing with your feet together, bend your left leg and take hold of its foot with your left hand. Stretch the front thigh muscles by pulling your foot as close to your seat as possible. Do not strain. Hold the position for 6 seconds before slowly releasing the leg to the floor. Bend the other leg, hold it with your other hand and stretch the muscles as before, holding the position for 6 seconds. Release your leg slowly to the floor.

THE WARM-UP AND AEROBIC WORKOUT

PREPARATORY STRETCHES

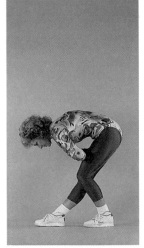

12 Hamstring stretch
Standing up straight, place one foot behind the other, keeping your feet hip-width apart and pointing straight ahead. Keep the front leg straight and bend the back leg, lowering your hips as much as possible without straining. Place your hands on your thigh (not on your knee) and hold the position for 6 seconds. Slowly straighten up then change the position of your legs and repeat the exercise with the other leg forwards, holding the position for 6 seconds. Slowly straighten up again.

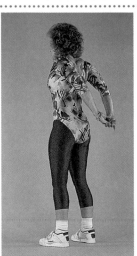

13 Chest and arm stretch
Standing with your feet hip-width apart and your knees slightly bent, slowly extend your hands behind your back and stretch your arms upwards. Do not interlink the fingers, just hold your hands together and extend your shoulders and your arms backwards as far as possible. Do not slump forwards. Hold the stretch position for 6 seconds then relax.

AEROBIC WORKOUT

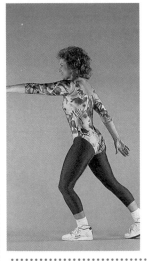

14 Low-impact spotty dog
Alternately step one foot backwards as you swing your opposite arm forwards. You should return to the central standing position between alternate steps. Move the arms in as big a movement as possible and continue for as long as is comfortable. This is a low-impact aerobic exercise, therefore one foot should always be on the floor.

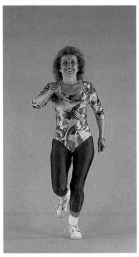

16 Jogging Jog on the spot for as many steps as is comfortable. Record your achievement and try to increase the number of steps next time you exercise.

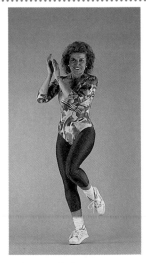

17 Step and clap Raising and bending alternate knees, step from side to side clapping your hands above shoulder level. Repeat as many times as is comfortable and record your achievement each time you exercise. Increase the number of repetitions as you become fitter.

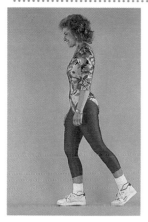

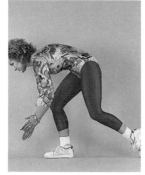

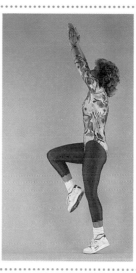

15 Clap low, clap high
Walk forwards for 3 steps

and then clap low, bending your knees and clapping your hands. Straighten up and walk backwards for 3 steps.

On the fourth step, skip and clap high above your head. Repeat this sequence 8 times, then repeat 8 times with the other leg forwards.

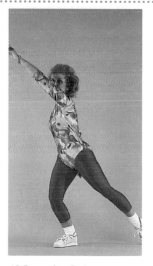

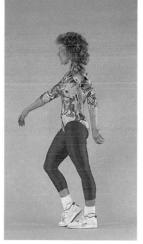

18 Lungeing Swing one arm across and upwards at the same time as stepping out sideways with the corresponding leg (e.g. right arm/right leg). Repeat to the other side with the other arm reaching across and the other leg stepping out. Repeat as many times as possible without straining.

19 Walking jog Walk on the spot, keeping your hands at a low level and repeat for 24 steps.

MUSCULAR STRENGTH AND ENDURANCE

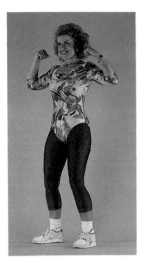

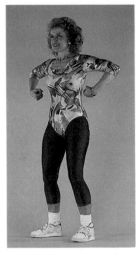

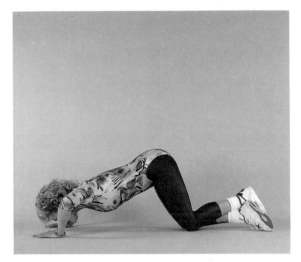

20 Bicep curl Standing with your feet hip-width apart and your knees slightly bent, make a fist with each hand and raise the arms to shoulder height. Bend the elbows, bringing your hands towards the shoulders, then straighten your arms out to your sides. Repeat the bending and straightening exercise 8 times.

21 Tricep curl With your arms still stretched out at shoulder level, bend them downwards with your fists towards your trunk. Straighten and bend your arms 8 times.

Now repeat the Bicep Curl and the Tricep Curl 8 more times.

22 Press-ups Position yourself on the floor on your hands and knees, placing your hands underneath your shoulders but set slightly wider apart. Place your knees slightly further back than hip level and cross your ankles. Slowly lower your head towards the floor, keeping your back as straight as possible, then raise up again. Repeat as many times as you can, increasing the number of repetitions as you become stronger. Do not strain. Record your progress each time you exercise.

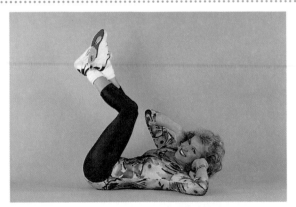

25 Waist whittler Lie on the floor with your knees slightly bent, cross your ankles and raise your legs. Place your hands to the sides of your head and raise your right shoulder towards your left knee to the count of 2. Then return to the floor to the count of 2. Repeat with left shoulder to right knee. Repeat 16 times (8 times to each alternate side).

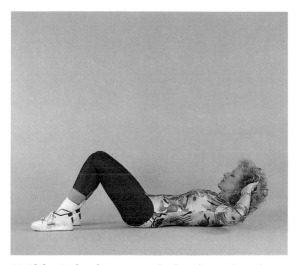

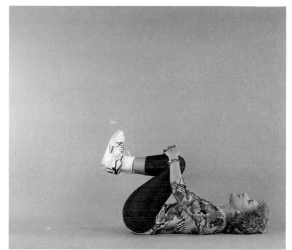

23 Abdominal curl Lie on your back with your knees bent and your feet flat on the floor. Place your hands to the sides of your head and slowly raise your head, shoulders and arms off the floor to the count of 2. Then lower your head, shoulders and arms to the floor to the count of 2. Breathe out as you raise your head and breathe in as you lower it. Repeat the exercise as many times as you can without straining, and record your progress each time you work out. Increase the number of repetitions as your tummy muscles become stronger.

24 Flex and point Lie on the floor, bend your knees and bring them towards your chest then place your hands around the front of your calves and flex both feet. Point the feet and continue flexing and then pointing. Feel the muscles in the front of your lower legs contracting as you flex your toes back. Repeat 8 times.

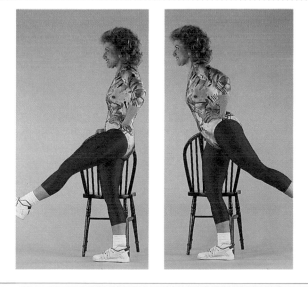

26 Hips and thighs Using a chair for support, swing one leg slowly forwards and backwards, keeping the standing leg slightly bent at the knee. Repeat the exercise with the same leg as many times as feels comfortable before turning round and repeating the exercise with the other leg. Record your progress and try to increase the number of repetitions each time you practise.

MUSCULAR STRENGTH AND ENDURANCE AND STRETCHES

STRENGTH AND ENDURANCE

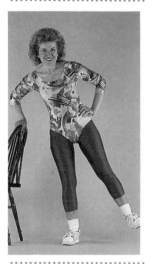

27 *Outer thighs* Again holding on to a chair, raise your outer leg straight out to the side ensuring that both feet are facing forwards. Slowly raise and lower the leg for as many repetitions as feels comfortable before turning round and repeating with the other leg. Record your progress and try to increase the number of repetitions each time you exercise.

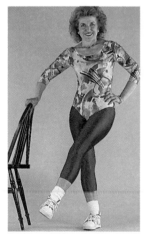

28 *Inner thighs* Hold on to a chair for support and stand on the leg nearest to the chair, with the knee slightly bent. Slowly bring the outer leg across as far as possible towards the chair. Slowly return it to its normal position and repeat the movement as many times as feels comfortable. You will be able to feel the muscle on the inner thigh working as you raise the outer leg across. Practise as many repetitions as you can before turning round and repeating the exercise with the other leg.

STRETCHES

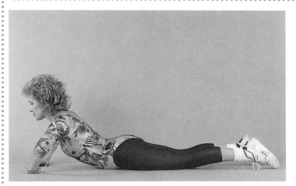

29 *Half cobra* Lie on your tummy on the floor and place your hands underneath your shoulders, fingers facing inwards. Slowly raise your head and shoulders off the floor, taking care not to straighten the arms completely. Feel the stretch down the central abdominal muscle. Hold in the extreme position for 8 seconds then slowly return to the floor.

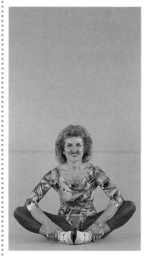

32 *Inner thigh stretch* Sitting with your knees apart and the soles of your feet placed together, place your elbows against your knees. Keeping your back straight, try to push your knees down without straining. Hold the position for 10 seconds and then, if you feel you can, push them down a little further and hold this position for another 10 seconds. Slowly relax and stand up.

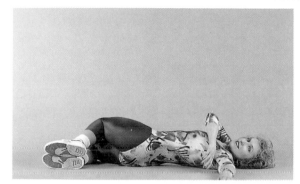

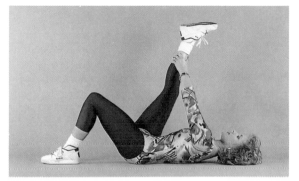

30 Waist and thigh stretch Roll over on to your back and bend your knees. Slowly allow your knees to drop down to the right side as you swing your arms over to the left side. Hold this gentle twist for the count of 10. Slowly straighten up and then twist to the other side and hold for the count of 10. Straighten up again.

31 Hamstring stretch Lying on your back with your knees bent and feet flat on the floor, slowly raise one knee towards your chest. Hold it with your hands for 8 seconds before straightening the leg and holding the calf or the thigh (whichever is more comfortable) in its stretched position but do not strain. Hold the position for 10 seconds and then, if you feel you can, slowly pull the leg towards you a little more and hold for a further 10 seconds. Then slowly bend the knee and return the foot to the floor. Repeat with the other leg but, again, do not strain.

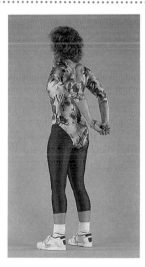

33 Chest and arm stretch Standing with your feet hip width apart and your knees slightly bent, slowly extend your hands behind your back, drawing your shoulders back as far as you can. Then raise your arms as high as possible, keeping them as straight as you can. Hold the stretch position for 8 seconds then slowly release.

REMOBILISE

To remobilise your body after this workout, please repeat Exercises 1, 2, 3, 4 and 5. Do as many repetitions as you feel is necessary to remobilise your joints and return your body to its pre-exercise state.

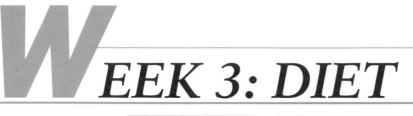

WEEK 3: DIET

You have now reached the halfway mark in this Whole Body Programme, and by now you should see a significant improvement in your figure. On the first day of week three weigh and measure yourself before you eat or drink anything. Enter the details on the Weight and Inch (Centimetre) Loss Record Chart on page 25. You may find your weight loss is not as dramatic this week. Now that you have settled into a new, healthier pattern of eating, your rate of weight loss will slow down as your level of fat decreases and your muscle tone increases. However, you may be pleasantly surprised by your inch loss, and remember it is what you see in the mirror that really counts.

DAY 15

BREAKFASTS
(R) 3 dried apricots (no-soak variety) chopped and mixed with 5 oz (125g) yogurt and ½ oz (12.5g) Branflakes
(B) 1 oz (25g) cereal plus 4 oz (100g) fresh fruit, finely chopped, plus milk from allowance and 1 teaspoon sugar
(V) 2 slices light bread spread with yogurt, filled with 1 sliced banana and 1 teaspoon preserve

LUNCHES
(R) 4 Ryvitas spread with 3 oz (75g) tinned tuna in brine, drained and mixed with 1 tablespoon yogurt and 1 tablespoon reduced-oil dressing, topped with cucumber
(B) Jacket potato (any size) topped with chopped onion mixed with 2 oz (50g) cottage cheese and 1 tablespoon reduced-oil dressing
(V) 1 lb (400g) fresh fruit plus 5 oz (125g) yogurt

DINNERS
(R) Fish Pie (see recipe, page 121), served with unlimited vegetables
(B) Blackeye Bean Casserole (see recipe, page 126), served with boiled rice
(V) Broccoli Delight (see recipe, page 127)

DAY 16

BREAKFASTS
(R) 4 oz (100g) stewed fruit, cooked without sugar, topped with 5 oz (125g) diet yogurt sprinkled with 1 oz (25g) sultanas pre-soaked in 1 tablespoon rum
(B) 1 piece any fresh fruit plus 1 slice toast spread with 2 teaspoons marmalade
(V) 6 apricots soaked overnight in hot tea, served with 5 oz (125g) natural yogurt

LUNCHES
(R) Prawn and Pasta Salad (see recipe, page 96), served with green salad
(B) 6 Ryvitas spread with Marmite and topped with 4 oz (100g) cottage cheese
(V) Cheesy Stuffed Potatoes (see recipe, page 91)

DINNERS
(R) Glazed Chicken (see recipe, page 116), served with unlimited vegetables
(B) Stir-fried Chicken and Vegetables (see recipe, page 119), served with boiled rice
(V) Chickpea and Fennel Casserole (see recipe, page 128), served with unlimited vegetables

DAY 17

BREAKFASTS
(R) 1 oz (25g) lean ham, grilled fresh tomatoes (unlimited quantity), 4 oz (100g) baked beans, 1 slice light bread, toasted
(B) 1½ oz (37.5g) any cereal with milk from allowance and 2 teaspoons sugar
(V) 6 oz (150g) stewed fruit, cooked without sugar, topped with 3 oz (75g) natural yogurt

LUNCHES
(R) Cheese, Prawn and Asparagus Salad (see recipe, page 90) plus 1 piece fresh fruit
(B) 1 wholemeal bread roll (approx. 2 oz/50g), spread with reduced-oil salad dressing and filled with salad, plus 1 piece fresh fruit
(V) Jacket potato (any size) topped with 1 oz (25g) sweetcorn mixed with 3 oz (75g) cottage cheese

DINNERS
(R) Hot Chicken Surprise (see recipe, page 117)
(B) Fish Curry (see recipe, page 121), served with boiled rice
(V) Tofu Burgers (see recipe, page 130), served with unlimited vegetables

DAY 18

BREAKFASTS
(R) 1 banana chopped and topped with 2 oz (50g) cottage cheese mixed with 1 tablespoon natural yogurt and 2 teaspoons raspberry jam
(B) 6 oz (150g) any stewed fruit, cooked without sugar
(V) 1 slice toast with 5 oz (125g) baked beans

LUNCHES
(R) 1 smoked trout (approx. 4 oz/100g) or 4 oz (100g) tinned tuna in brine (drained), served with mixed salad plus dressing of 2 oz (50g) natural yogurt mixed with 1 teaspoon horseradish sauce
(B) Beef and Vegetable Soup (see recipe, page 100) plus 1 slice toast
(V) Jacket potato with Ratatouille (see recipe, page 135)

DINNERS
(R) Beefburgers (see recipe, page 103), served with Oven Chips (see recipe, page 134), mushrooms, peas and sweetcorn
(B) Lamb Stew (see recipe, page 104)
(V) Vegetable and Fruit Curry (see recipe, page 130), served with boiled rice

DAY 19

BREAKFASTS
(R) 5 prunes in natural juice, served with ½ oz (12.5g) any cereal and 1 tablespoon yogurt
(B) 1 oz (25g) any cereal, with ¼ pint (125ml) milk in addition to allowance and 1 oz (25g) sultanas
(V) 1 oz (25g) any cereal mixed with 5 oz (125g) yogurt and grated apple

LUNCHES
(R) Jacket potato topped with 2 oz (50g) smoked mackerel fillet flaked and mixed with 1 oz (25g) each sweetcorn and peas and 1 tablespoon reduced-oil dressing and 1 tablespoon yogurt
(B) Triple-decker sandwich (3 slices light bread spread with Marmite and reduced-oil dressing, filled with 2 oz [50g] cottage cheese and salad)
(V) ½ pint (250ml) Minestrone Soup (see recipe, page 102) plus 1 wholemeal roll

DINNERS
(R) Cold Prawn and Rice Salad (see recipe, page 120)
(B) Niçoise Salad (see recipe, page 122)
(V) Vegetarian Loaf (see recipe, page 132)

DAY 20

BREAKFASTS
(R) 2 bananas, sliced and topped with 1 raspberry 'petit' fromage frais
(B) 1½ oz (37.5g) any cereal, with ¼ pint (5 fl oz/125ml) milk in addition to allowance and 1 teaspoon sugar
(V) 1 slice toast spread with 1 teaspoon jam any flavour, topped with 3 oz (75g) cottage cheese

LUNCHES
(R) Kiwifruit and Ham Open Sandwich (see recipe, page 94)
(B) 1 slice toast spread with Marmite and topped with 1 poached egg
(V) Jacket potato (any size) topped with 4 oz (100g) baked beans

DINNERS
(R) Marinaded Lamb (see recipe, page 105) with Lemon Glazed Vegetables (see recipe, page 135)
(B) Lambs Liver with Orange (see recipe, page 104), served with unlimited vegetables
(V) Sweetcorn and Potato Fritters (see recipe, page 129), served with Ratatouille (see recipe, page 135)

DAY 21

BREAKFASTS
(R) 2 pieces any fresh fruit plus 2 × 5 oz (2 × 125g) diet yogurts, any flavour
(B) Porridge (see recipe, page 90)
(V) Banana Milk Shake (see recipe, page 89)

LUNCHES
(R) Jacket potato (6–8 oz/150–200g) topped with 3 oz (75g) tinned tuna in brine, drained, flaked and mixed with chopped cucumber and 1 tablespoon reduced-oil salad dressing and 1 tablespoon natural yogurt seasoned with 1 teaspoon lemon juice, salt and black pepper
(B) 4 pieces any fresh fruit
(V) 2 slices bread spread with Marmite and filled with 3 oz (75g) cottage cheese and salad, plus 1 piece fruit

DINNERS
(R) Ham, Beef and Chicken Salad (see recipe, page 104)
(B) Barbecued Pork Kebabs (see recipe for Barbecued Kebabs, page 102), served with boiled rice mixed with beansprouts
(V) Oat and Cheese Loaf (see recipe, page 129)

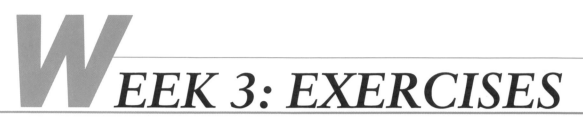

WARM-UP I: MOBILISER

I hope you managed to progress through last week's workout programme. This week we work our body a little harder and some of the exercises have been changed to make them more difficult. If you find yourself struggling with the new exercises, replace them with the easier versions from earlier weeks until you feel you are able to progress to this week's exercises without straining. It is better to do an easier exercise properly than a more advanced one incorrectly.

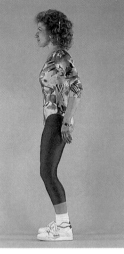

1 Shoulder rolls Standing with your feet hip-width apart and your knees slightly bent, slowly roll both shoulders simultaneously backwards 8 times, and then roll them forwards 8 times. Repeat both movements again 8 times.

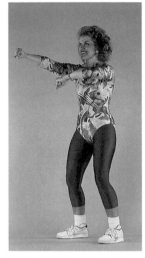

2 Punching Standing with your feet comfortably apart, knees slightly bent and tummy pulled in, raise your arms to shoulder level in front and punch forwards with alternate arms. Repeat 16 times (8 for each hand).

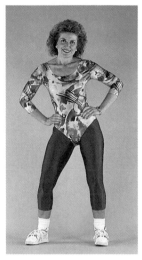

3 Pelvic rotation With your hands on your hips, rotate your hips 4 times in a clockwise direction and then 4 times in an anti-clockwise direction. Repeat this movement with 4 more rotations in each direction.

WARM-UP III: PREPARATORY STRETCHES

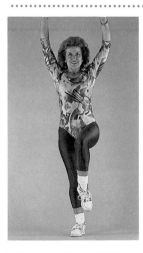

7 Marching, arm raising Marching on the spot with big leg movements, raise your arms out to the sides and up above your head then down again as you place each foot back on the floor. Do as many steps as you can comfortably and increase the number of repetitions as you become fitter. Record your progress each time you work out.

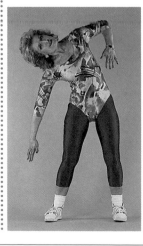

8 Waist stretch Standing with your feet apart and knees slightly bent, slowly curve your spine sideways and hold the position for 8 seconds. Slowly straighten up then curve over to the other side and hold for 8 seconds. Relax.

THE WARM-UP

WARM-UP II: PULSE RAISER

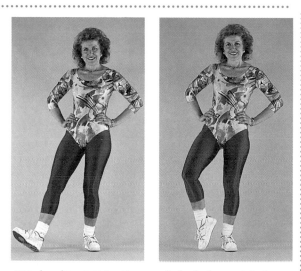

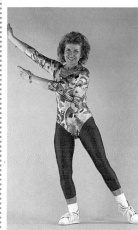

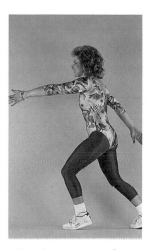

4 Heel and toe tapping First tap the heel of your right foot and then the toe. Repeat 8 times (8 heels and 8 toes) then repeat with your left foot.

5 Swing and point Swinging your arms gently from side to side, move your weight on to alternate feet and point the foot of the straight leg. Repeat 16 times (8 to each side).

6 Low-impact spotty dog Alternately swing one arm forwards as you step back with the opposite foot. You should return to the central standing position between alternate steps. Move the arms in as big a movement as possible and repeat the exercise as many times as you can comfortably, increasing with fitness. Record your progress.

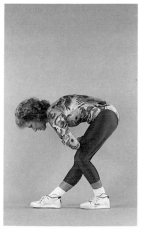

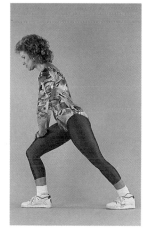

9 Hamstring stretch Standing up straight, place one foot behind the other, keeping your feet hip-width apart and pointing straight ahead. Keep the front leg straight and bend the back leg, lowering your hips as much as possible without straining. Place your hands on your thigh (not on your knee) and hold the position for 8 seconds. Slowly straighten up. Proceed to the next exercise.

10 Calf stretch Step back further with the back leg and, keeping it straight and with the back heel flat on the floor, bend your front knee. Keeping both feet pointing straight ahead and ensuring the heel of the back foot remains flat on the floor, bend the front knee forwards over your foot. Do not strain. Hold the position for 8 seconds then slowly straighten up.

Repeat Exercises 9 and 10 with the other leg in front.

THE WARM-UP AND AEROBIC WORKOUT

PREPARATORY STRETCHES

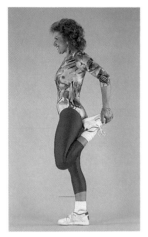

11 Front thigh stretch Bend your left leg and take hold of its foot with your left hand. Pull your foot close to your seat. Do not strain. Hold for the count of 8, feeling the stretch down the front of your thigh. Slowly release. Repeat with the other leg.

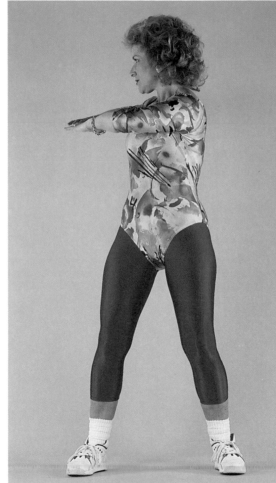

12 Waist twist Stand with your feet hip-width apart and your knees slightly bent. Raise your arms to shoulder level in front and bend your elbows so they point out to the sides. Slowly twist your upper body to one side then hold the extreme position for 10 seconds. Slowly return to the central position and twist to the other side and hold the extreme position for 10 seconds.

AEROBIC WORKOUT

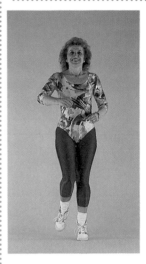

13 Jogging Jog on the spot for as many steps as you feel is comfortable. Record the number of steps and try to increase the number each time you practise.

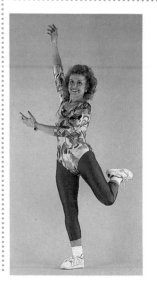

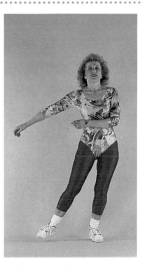

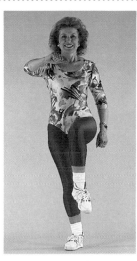

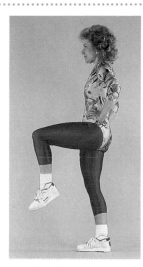

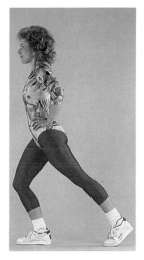

14 *Sideways jogging*
Allowing your arms to swing with you, jog sideways. Count the number of steps that you can do without discomfort and record your progress. Increase the number of steps with practice.

15 *Marching on the spot*
March on the spot swinging your arms as you step. Make the leg movements as big as possible and ensure that you place the heel down each time you step on to the floor. Repeat as many times as you can comfortably and record your progress.

16 *Lift and step* Raise your left knee then lower it and extend it out behind you.

Repeat this movement 8 times with your left leg and then repeat with your right leg.

17 *Swing and kick* Swing your arms first in front and then as high as possible to one side and at the same time allow the opposite leg to bend in a back-kick movement. Return the bent leg to the floor then swing your arms to the other side, lifting the other leg behind. Practise so that you get into the momentum of the exercise and repeat 16 times (8 to each side). As you become fitter you can skip as you do it. Record your progress each time you exercise.

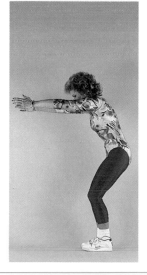

18 *Ski down* Stand with your feet hip-width apart and your hands by your sides. Pulling your tummy in, raise your hands above your head and gently swing them down by your sides as you bend your knees. Slowly reach up as you straighten again and repeat the exercise 12 times.

MUSCULAR STRENGTH AND ENDURANCE

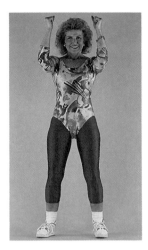 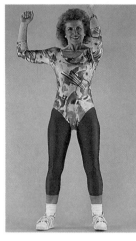 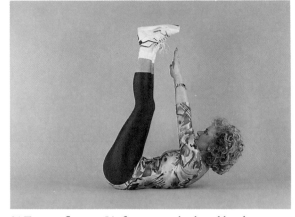

19 Chest expander Bend your elbows and make a fist with each hand. Bring your arms forwards in front of your face then out again to the sides. Repeat 8 times.

20 Chest expander (singles) Remain in a similar position to the last exercise but this time bring only one arm forwards and back. Repeat 8 times with each arm.

21 Tummy flattener Lie flat on your back and bend your knees towards your chest. Raise your legs straight up. Slowly raise your head and shoulders off the floor to the count of 5, raising your arms and pointing your fingers towards your toes. Lower your head and shoulders to the count of 5. Breathe out as you raise up and breathe in as you lower to the floor. Repeat 4 times at first and increase the number of repetitions as you become fitter.

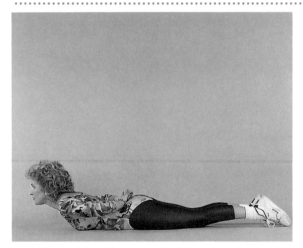 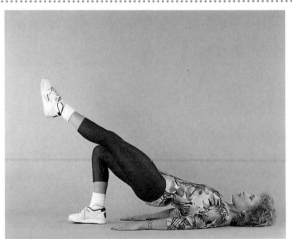

24 Back strengthener Lie on your tummy on the floor and place your hands (palms upwards) in the small of your back. Slowly raise your head and shoulders off the floor to the count of 3 then slowly lower back to the floor to the count of 3. Repeat 4 times at first but try to increase the number of repetitions as you get fitter. Record your progress each time you work out.

25 Hip lifter Lie on your back with your knees bent, your feet flat on the floor and your hands by your sides. Extend your left leg so that it is parallel with the thigh of your right leg then slowly raise your hips off the floor and slowly lower again. Repeat 8 times to begin with. As you become stronger you can hold the elevated position and move your left leg up and down about 2 inches (5 cm) 8 times before lowering your hips to the floor and bending the leg. Repeat to the other side. Don't try to do too much on the first attempt at this exercise; take it very gently and slowly.

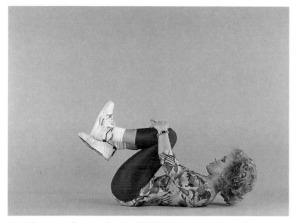

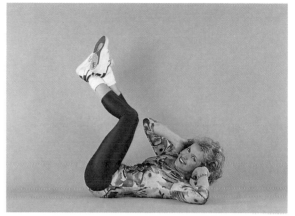

22 Alternate flex and point Still lying on the floor, bend your knees towards your chest and place your hands around the front of your calves. Alternately flex and point your feet and feel the front calf muscles working as you flex your toes back. Point and flex each foot 12 times. Record your progress and try to increase the number of repetitions as you become fitter.

23 Waist whittler Lie on your back on the floor and raise your legs towards the ceiling, keeping them slightly bent, and cross your ankles. Place your hands to the sides of your head and raise your right shoulder towards your left raised knee to the count of 2. Lower to the count of 2. Breathe out as you raise up and breathe in as you lower down. Repeat with the other shoulder. Repeat with alternate shoulders 16 times (8 to each side), then repeat again.

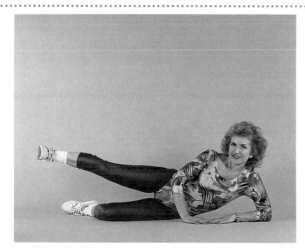

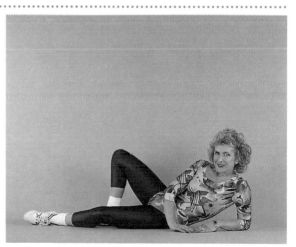

26 Outer thigh streamliner Lie on your left side and prop yourself up on your elbow. Bend your left leg and ensure that you keep your body in a straight line throughout this exercise. Extend your right leg, flex your foot and raise the leg about 12 inches (30 cm). Lower it again, controlling the movement to avoid jerkiness. Repeat the lift 16 times at first, increasing the number of repetitions as you get fitter. Proceed to the next exercise.

27 Inner thigh streamliner Bend your right leg and place its foot behind your left knee. Extend the left leg and raise it off the floor as far as possible without straining. This will only be 3-4 inches (7.5-10 cm). Lower your leg and repeat the exercise as many times as feels comfortable.

Roll over on to your right side and repeat Exercises 26 and 27, increasing the number of repetitions as you become fitter.

STRETCHES

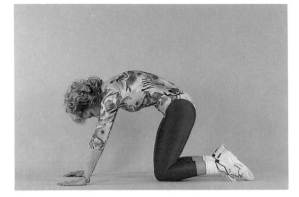

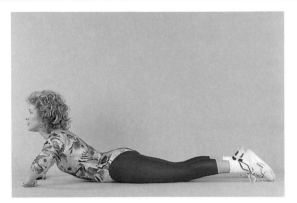

28 Back curl Place yourself on your hands and knees with your hands shoulder-width apart. Curl your pelvis forwards and arch your spine. Hold this position for 10 seconds then slowly relax.

29 Half cobra Lie on your tummy on the floor and place your hands underneath your chin with the fingers facing inwards. Slowly raise your head and shoulders off the floor but do not straighten your arms and do not raise very far. Hold for 10 seconds then slowly return to the floor.

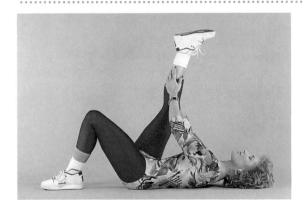

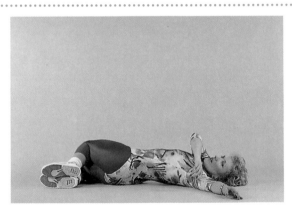

31 Hamstring stretch With both knees bent and feet flat on the floor, bring one knee up towards your chest and then extend the leg as far as possible. Take hold of your calf or your thigh (not behind the knee) and hold the position to the count of 10. If, after that, you feel you are able to bring your leg further forwards, do so and hold for a further 10 seconds. Slowly lower the extended leg back to the floor then repeat with the other leg.

32 Waist and thigh stretch Lie on the floor with your hands stretched out to the sides, your knees bent, and your feet flat on the floor. Slowly allow your knees to drop to the right side and bring your hands over to the left so that you twist at the waist. Hold this position for 10 seconds then slowly return to the starting position. Repeat by twisting to the other side.

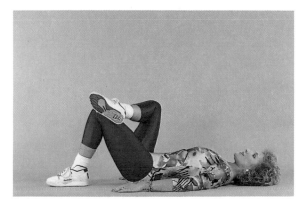

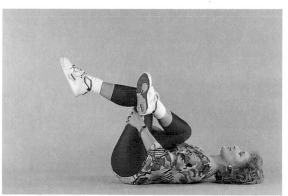

30 Corkscrew Lie on your back with your knees bent, feet flat on the floor, and your hands by your sides. Place your right leg in front of the left knee. Slowly raise your left leg, place your hands around the back of its thigh and pull it towards you. Keep your head and shoulders on the floor.

Feel the stretch in the large muscle around your hips. Hold the position for 10 seconds then slowly return both feet to the floor. Place your left leg in front of the right knee and repeat the exercise with this leg forwards.

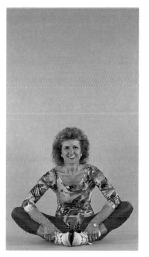

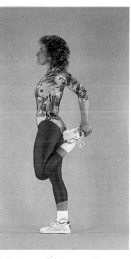

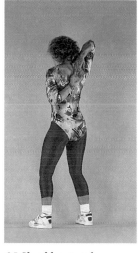

33 Inner thigh stretch
Sitting with your knees apart and the soles of your feet placed together, rest your elbows against your knees. Keeping your back straight, try to push your knees down without straining. Hold the position for 10 seconds and then, if you can, try to push your knees down a little further and hold for another 10 seconds. Slowly relax then stand up.

34 Front thigh stretch
Standing with your feet together, bend your left leg and take hold of the foot with your left hand. Stretch the front thigh muscles by pulling your foot as close to your seat as possible. Do not strain. Hold the position for 6 seconds before slowly releasing the leg to the floor. Repeat with your right leg.

35 Shoulder stretch
Standing with your feet hip-width apart and your knees slightly bent, bring your right arm up over your head and down your back while bringing your left arm up behind your back. Clasp your fingers together if possible and hold the extreme position for 10 seconds. Slowly release then repeat the exercise reversing the position of the arms.

REMOBILISE

To remobilise your body after this workout, please repeat Exercises 1, 2, 3, 4 and 5. Do as many repetitions as you feel is necessary to remobilise your joints and leave your body feeling revitalised.

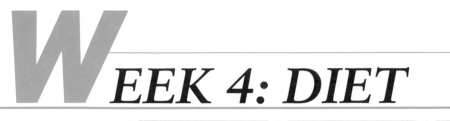

WEEK 4: DIET

This is the final week of the programme – did you think you would ever get this far? Check your progress in the mirror and see the transformation to date. Don't forget to weigh and measure yourself and enter the details on the Weight and Inch (Centimetre) Loss Record Chart on page 25. By the end of this week you will see the incredible results you have achieved.

DAY 22

BREAKFASTS
(**R**) 8 oz (200g) fresh fruit salad topped with 1 'petit' fromage frais
(**B**) 1 slice toast spread with 1 teaspoon jam and topped with 1 small banana, mashed
(**V**) 1 egg scrambled without butter on 1 slice toast spread with Marmite, and topped with 5 oz (125g) tinned tomatoes

LUNCHES
(**R**) 5 Ryvitas spread with 2 oz (50g) tinned salmon in brine mixed with 2 oz (50g) cottage cheese and 1 tablespoon reduced-oil salad dressing
(**B**) 4 slices light bread spread with Marmite, filled with 1 sliced hard-boiled egg and sliced tomatoes
(**V**) Courgette and Tomato Salad (see recipe, page 92)

DINNERS
(**R**) Indian Chicken (see recipe, page 117), served with unlimited vegetables
(**B**) Vegetarian Goulash (see recipe, page 132), served with boiled brown rice
(**V**) Tikka Lentil Bake (see recipe, page 80)

DAY 23

BREAKFASTS
(**R**) 3 green figs plus 5 oz (125g) diet yogurt
(**B**) 2 oz (50g) any cereal, milk from allowance and 1 teaspoon sugar
(**V**) 4 oz (100g) cottage cheese mixed with 1 tablespoon jam or honey

LUNCHES
(**R**) Oriental Stir-fry (see recipe, page 95)
(**B**) 3 slices light bread, toasted, topped with 5 oz (125g) baked beans and 8 oz (200g) tinned tomatoes boiled and reduced to a creamy consistency
(**V**) Chilli Salad (see recipe, page 91)

DINNERS
(**R**) Poached Trout with Cucumber Sauce (see recipe, page 123), served with green salad
(**B**) Chicken Fricassée (see recipe, page 112), served with unlimited vegetables
(**V**) Creamy Horseradish and Watercress Crumble (see recipe, page 86)

DAY 24

BREAKFASTS
(**R**) 8 oz (200g) seedless grapes mixed with 8 oz (200g) chopped melon and 5 oz (125g) yogurt
(**B**) 8 oz (200g) stewed fruit, cooked without sugar, plus ⅛ pint (2 fl oz/50ml) milk in addition to allowance
(**V**) 5 prunes in natural juice mixed with ½ oz (12.5g) Branflakes and 1 tablespoon natural yogurt

LUNCHES
(**R**) 1-egg omelette, cooked without oil in a non-stick frying pan, filled with 2 oz (50g) low-fat fromage frais mixed with sliced boiled mushrooms and chopped green peppers, and served with a large salad
(**B**) 4 slices light bread spread with Marmite and filled with 2 oz (50g) cottage cheese plus grated carrot
(**V**) Oat and Cheese Loaf (see recipe, page 95)

DINNERS
(**R**) Chinese Chicken Salad (see recipe, page 116)
(**B**) Potato Madras (see recipe, page 129)
(**V**) Three-Layer Millet Bake (see recipe, page 84)

DAY 25

BREAKFASTS
(R) 2 slices light bread spread with mustard or other permitted sauce and 2 rashers lean bacon (all fat removed), grilled
(B) 1 wholemeal bread roll (approx. 2 oz/50g) spread with 2 teaspoons jam, honey or marmalade
(V) 8 oz (200g) stewed fruit, cooked without sugar, plus 1 oz (25g) sultanas, served with 5 oz (125g) diet yogurt

LUNCHES
(R) Chicken and Mushroom Soup (see recipe page 100)
(B) 8 oz (200g) Coleslaw (see recipe, page 133) plus 4 oz (100g) baked beans, and salad
(V) Triple-decker sandwich made with 3 slices light bread spread with reduced-oil salad dressing and filled with 2 oz (50g) cottage cheese and salad

DINNERS
(R) Rosy Duck Salad (see recipe, page 118)
(B) Chicken and Potato Cakes (see recipe, page 111), served with unlimited vegetables
(V) Chickpea Couscous (see recipe, page 88)

DAY 26

BREAKFASTS
(R) 1 oz (25g) Branflakes and 1 oz (25g) sultanas with ¼ pint (5 fl oz/125ml) milk from allowance
(B) 2 pieces any fresh fruit plus 1 slice toast spread with 1 teaspoon marmalade
(V) 1 oz (25g) muesli (any brand) plus 2 no-soak apricots, chopped, served with ¼ pint (5 fl oz/125ml) milk in addition to allowance

LUNCHES
(R) 4 Ryvitas topped with Spring Salad (see recipe, page 97)
(B) Creamy Vegetable Soup (see recipe, page 101) plus 1 slice light bread
(V) Cheese and Apricot Pears (see recipe, page 90)

DINNERS
(R) Coq au Vin (see recipe, page 114), served with boiled potatoes
(B) Cottage Pie (see recipe, page 128), served with unlimited vegetables
(V) Tofu Indonesian Style (see recipe, page 81)

DAY 27

BREAKFASTS
(R) 8 oz (200g) smoked haddock, cooked in milk in addition to allowance
(B) 8 oz (200g) stewed rhubarb, cooked without sugar, topped with ⅛ pint (2 fl oz/50ml) milk in addition to allowance, plus 1 slice toast spread with 1 teaspoon marmalade
(V) 1 boiled or poached egg on 1 slice toast spread with Marmite

LUNCHES
(R) 4 oz (100g) cold cooked chicken, served with Spinach and Mushroom Salad (see recipe, page 133)
(B) ½ pint (10 fl oz/250ml) Chicken Soup (see recipe, page 100) plus 4 Ryvitas spread with Marmite
(V) 4 oz (100g) baked beans and 4 oz (100g) tinned spaghetti in tomato sauce, served with 2 slices toast

DINNERS
(R) Stir-fried Chicken and Vegetables (see recipe, page 119), served with boiled rice
(B) Curried Chicken and Yogurt Salad (see recipe, page 94)
(V) Hearty Hotpot (see recipe, page 128)

DAY 28

BREAKFASTS
(R) Pineapple Boat (see recipe, page 90)
(B) 1 slice toast topped with 8 oz (200g) baked beans
(V) 1½ oz (37.5g) muesli (any brand) with ¼ pint (5 fl oz/125ml) milk in addition to allowance

LUNCHES
(R) Chilli Bacon Potatoes (see recipe, page 91)
(B) Mixed Vegetable Soup (see recipe, page 102) and 1 slice bread
(V) Chinese Apple Salad (see recipe, page 92) plus 2 oz (50g) cottage cheese

DINNERS
(R) Chicken and Mushroom Pilaff (see recipe, page 110)
(B) Chicken and Potato Pie (see recipe, page 111), served with unlimited vegetables (excluding additional potatoes)
(V) Vegetable Mirepoix in Filo Overcoat (see recipe, page 82)

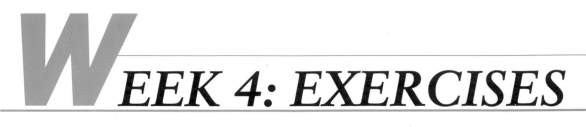
WARM-UP I: MOBILISER

If you have managed to do the workouts so far, pat yourself on the back! You must be feeling significantly fitter and your shape will already be improved. Just one more week to go and in this week's programme I have included some fairly advanced exercises designed for those who have worked out daily over the last 3 weeks. Only do what you can without straining and, if necessary, replace these exercises with alternatives from previous weeks.

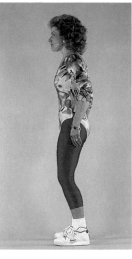

1 Shoulder rotation Standing with your feet slightly apart and your knees slightly bent, rotate both shoulders backwards 8 times and then forwards 8 times. Repeat 8 times more in each direction.

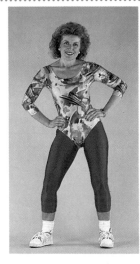

2 Pelvic rotation With hands placed on your hips, rotate your hips 4 times in a clockwise direction and then 4 times in an anti-clockwise direction. Repeat this movement for 4 rotations in each direction.

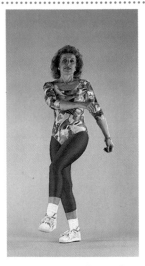

3 Arm swinging, knee raises Swinging your arms gently from side to side, raise alternate knees across your body. Repeat 16 times (8 for each leg).

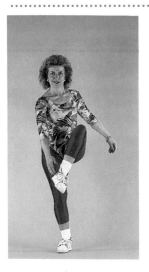

7 Alternate foot raises Raise one foot towards the opposite hand and attempt a small jump as you do so. Repeat with the other foot and continue this skipping movement for as many times as you can without discomfort. Increase the number of repetitions as you become fitter.

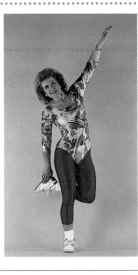

8 Kick and touch Swinging your left arm as high as possible, kick your left leg behind the right one and touch your left foot with your right hand. Repeat, exercising the opposite arm and leg. When you have mastered this exercise you may be able to add a jump to your step to give a greater aerobic benefit. Repeat the exercise as many times as you can without discomfort. Record your progress and try to increase the number of repetitions as you become fitter.

THE WARM-UP

WARM-UP II: PULSE RAISER

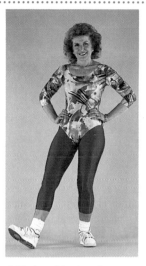

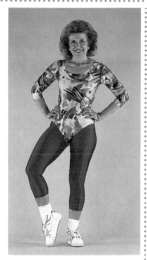

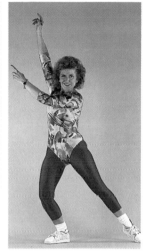

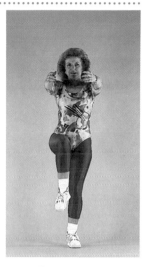

4 Heel and toe tapping
With hands on your hips, first tap the heel of one foot

and then tap the toe. Repeat 8 times (8 heels and 8 toes) and then repeat with the other foot. Repeat the whole exercise again with each foot.

5 Swing and point Swinging your arms across your body to the right as high as possible, extend your left leg out to the side and point the toe. Then swing your arms in the opposite direction. Repeat as many swings as you can comfortably.

6 Marching, arms out and in Marching on the spot with large steps, take your arms out to the sides and then into the centre in front of your chest. Repeat as many times as you can comfortably. Record your progress.

WARM-UP III: PREPARATORY STRETCHES

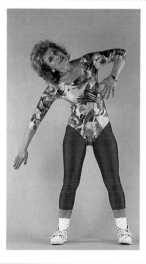

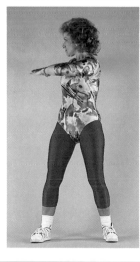

9 Waist stretch Standing with your knees slightly bent, slowly curve your spine over sideways and hold the position for 8 seconds. Slowly straighten up and then curve over to the other side and hold the position for 8 seconds. Straighten up and relax.

10 Waist twist Stand with your feet apart and knees slightly bent. Raise your arms to shoulder level in front and bend your elbows so they point out to the sides. Slowly twist the upper body to one side and hold the position for 8 seconds. Slowly return to the central position and then twist to the opposite side and hold the position for 8 seconds. Slowly return to the central position and relax.

THE WARM-UP AND AEROBIC WORKOUT

PREPARATORY STRETCHES

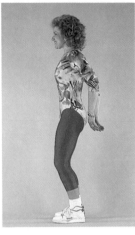

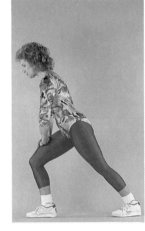

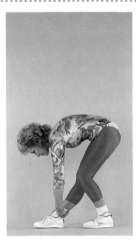

11 *Chest stretch* Standing with your knees slightly bent and your arms hanging by your sides, draw your shoulders back stretching the muscles across your upper chest. Hold for 6 seconds then relax.

12 *Calf stretch* Stand with your feet hip-width apart and one foot behind the other. Ensuring that the back heel remains flat on the floor, bend the front leg and lean forwards placing your hand on your thigh. Hold the stretch position for 8 seconds then straighten up. Change the position of your legs so that the other leg is now in front and repeat the exercise. Straighten up and relax.

13 *Hamstring stretch* Stand with your feet hip-width apart and one foot placed closely behind the other. Keeping your front leg straight, slowly bend your back leg. Place your hands around your calf or your ankle, whichever is most comfortable, and hold the extreme position for 8 seconds. Relax and straighten up. Change the position of your legs and repeat with the other leg.

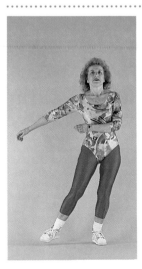

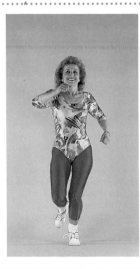

16 *Sideways jogging* Jog from side to side, allowing your arms to swing with you. Repeat as many times as possible and record the number of repetitions.

17 *Jogging* Jog on the spot, swinging your arms as you do so. Continue for as many steps as you wish, according to your level of fitness. Record your progress each time you exercise.

AEROBIC WORKOUT

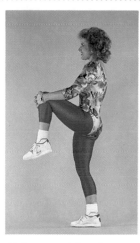

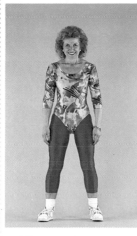

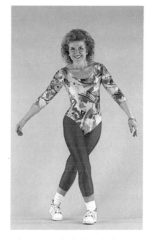

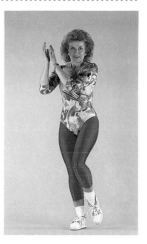

14 *Seat stretch* Standing on your right leg, bring your left knee towards your chest and hold your left leg with your hands. Hold the position for 10 seconds and feel the stretch in the muscle from your seat. Relax then repeat with your right leg.

15 *The grapevine* Remember this is a 3-steps-and-a-skip movement. Standing with your feet comfortably apart, step out sideways with your right foot.

Place your left foot behind your right one, then step out again with your right foot. Finish with a skip and a clap. Repeat the movement in the opposite direction. Move your arms in a breaststroke motion as you step sideways.

Repeat this sequence of movements in between the following four high-impact aerobic exercises. To do so will enable you to keep your pulse rate high without becoming over-tired.

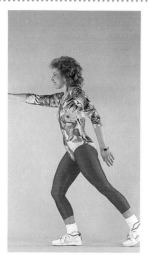

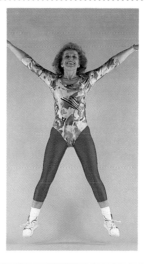

18 *Spotty dog* In a single movement jump back with your left leg and swing your right arm forwards. Then jump the opposite way with your right leg back and your left arm forwards. Continue this movement for as many repetitions as you can do comfortably. Record your progress and increase the number of repetitions as you become fitter.

19 *Jumping jacks* Stand with your feet together and your arms by your sides. Jump so that you land with your feet apart and your hands high. As you land on the floor ensure your knees bend over your ankles and not inwards. Jump again, lowering your hands to your sides and bringing your feet together into the starting position, bending your knees slightly as you land. This exercise should be performed rhythmically, jumping out and in, in time with the music. Repeat the movement as many times as you wish.

MUSCULAR STRENGTH AND ENDURANCE

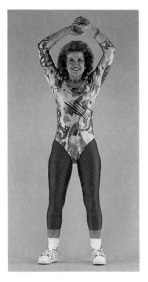

20 *Arm lifts* Standing with your feet hip-width apart and your knees slightly bent, extend your arms out to your sides (like a scarecrow) then raise them above your head, bending them slightly. Keeping your arms bent, lower them to shoulder level, and then raise them again. Repeat 16 times. Rest for a moment by swinging your arms in front of you and then raise them again to do another 16 shoulder raises.

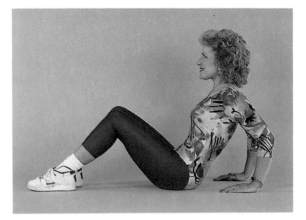

21 *Tricep dip* Sit on the floor with your knees bent and your feet flat on the floor. Place your hands behind you with your fingers pointing forwards. Bend your arms and slowly raise your body up and down, working the muscles in the backs of your arms. Do not allow your elbows to lock when you sit up. Repeat as many times as you can without discomfort. Keep a record of your progress.

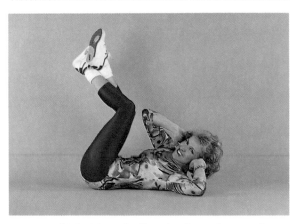

24 *Waist whittler* Lie on the floor, bend your knees and raise your legs towards the ceiling, crossing the ankles. Twist your right shoulder up towards your left knee to the count of 3 then slowly uncurl to the count of 3. Breathe out as you curl up and breathe in as you lower yourself down. Repeat with the left shoulder raised towards your right knee. Repeat as many times as you can without discomfort and record your progress each time you exercise.

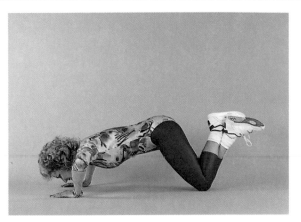

25 *Press-ups* If you have coped easily with the press-ups so far, see if you can progress to this more advanced version. Position yourself on your hands and knees and place your hands further apart than the width of your shoulders and your knees further back than your hips. Cross your ankles and raise your feet off the floor. Bend your elbows and lower yourself towards the floor and raise up again as many times as you can without discomfort. Keep a record of your progress and aim to increase the number of repetitions each time you practise.

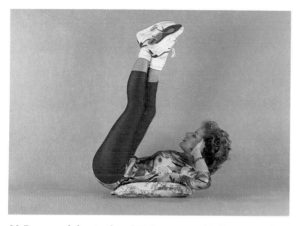

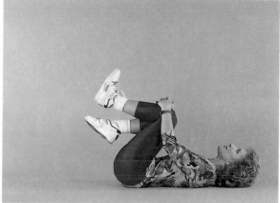

22 Reverse abdominal curl Only attempt this if you can do the earlier abdominal exercises easily. You may find the use of a cushion helpful during this exercise. Lie on the floor, bend your knees slightly, raise your legs and cross your ankles. Place your hands at the sides of your head then slowly raise your head and shoulders and, at the same time, raise your hips off the floor to the count of 3. Lower to the count of 3. Breathe out as you raise and in as you lower.

23 Alternate flex and point This exercise works the front of your calves. Lie on your back, cuddle your knees and alternately flex and point each foot in turn. Repeat this movement as many times as you wish between sets of repetitions of the *Reverse abdominal curl* (Exercise 22). It allows your abdominal muscles to relax and recover between repetitions of the previous exercise.

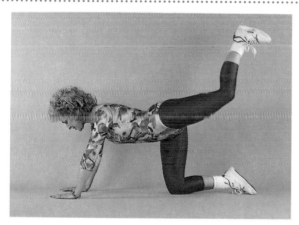

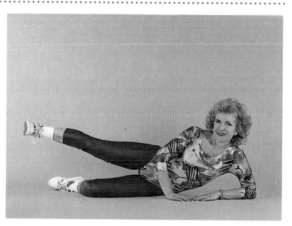

26 Bottom lifter Position yourself on your hands and knees and place your hands shoulder-width apart, fingers facing forwards. Raise one leg, with the foot flexed, straight out behind you so that it is in line with the rest of your body, then bend it and push the heel of your foot towards the ceiling. Repeat this small lifting movement, keeping your foot flexed throughout, as many times as you can without discomfort. Change position and repeat with the other leg as many times as possible. Record your progress and try to increase the number of repetitions as your muscles become stronger.

27 Outer thigh streamliner Lie on your left side, either propping yourself up on your elbow or lying with your arm outstretched above your head. Bend your left leg but keep your right leg extended. Keep the knee and hips facing forwards at all times. Raise your right leg up and down about 12 inches (30 cm), keeping it as straight as possible. Control the movement to avoid jerkiness. Repeat it as many times as you can comfortably and record your progress. Proceed to the next exercise before turning over on to your right side.

MUSCULAR STRENGTH AND ENDURANCE

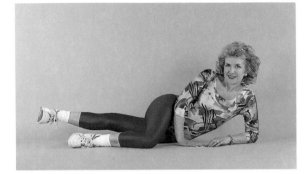

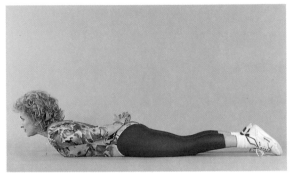

28 Inner thigh streamliner Bend your right leg and place it in front of your left leg, which should be extended straight. Flex the foot of your left leg and try to raise it up and down as far as possible. This is likely to be only 3-4 inches (7.5-10 cm). Feel the inner thigh muscle of the straight leg working as you raise and lower it. Repeat as many lifts as possible without straining. Roll over on to your right side and repeat Exercises 27 and 28 working your left leg.

29 Back strengthener Roll over on to your front and place your hands in the small of your back. Slowly raise your head and shoulders off the floor to the count of 4 then slowly lower them to the count of 4. Repeat the exercise as many times as you can without discomfort. Record the number of repetitions each time you work out.

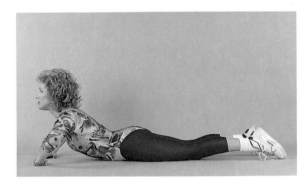

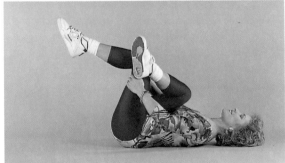

32 Half cobra Lie on your tummy on the floor and place your hands underneath your chin with the fingers facing inwards. Slowly raise your head and shoulders off the floor but do not go very far. Do *not* attempt to straighten the arms or hunch your shoulders. Hold the position for 8 seconds then slowly lower yourself to the floor.

33 Corkscrew Lie on your back with your knees bent, your feet flat on the floor and your hands by your sides. Raise your right leg in front of the left knee. Slowly raise the left leg and place your hands around the back of the thigh and pull it towards you. Keep your head and shoulders on the floor. Feel the stretch in the large muscle around your hips. Hold the position for the count of 10 then slowly return both feet to the floor. Repeat with the left leg raised.

34 Hamstring stretch Lie on your back, bend both knees and place feet flat on the floor. Slowly bring one leg up towards your chest and then extend it as far as possible without overstretching your hamstrings. Take hold of your calf or your thigh (not behind the knee) and hold the position for 10 seconds. Then, if possible, stretch the leg forwards a little further and hold for another 10 seconds. Slowly bend and lower the leg back to the floor then repeat with the other leg. (See page 64).

STRETCHES

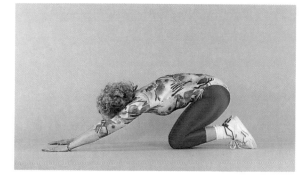

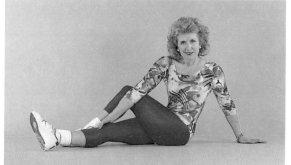

30 Cat stretch Position yourself on your hands and knees and slowly lean back towards your feet without allowing your seat to rest on your heels. Stretch out your arms as far as possible and enjoy the beautiful stretch throughout your body. Hold the extreme position for 10 seconds then relax.

31 Body twister Sit as shown. Place your left leg over your right leg so that it rests on the far side of your right knee. Bring your right arm forwards so that its elbow is by your left knee and your right hand is on your right knee. Slowly twist around to your left and place your left hand beside or behind you. Slowly twist your body away from your legs and hold for 10 seconds. Return to the starting position and then repeat to the other side.

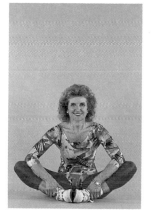

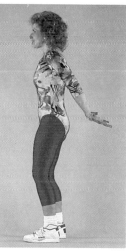

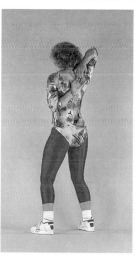

35 Inner thigh stretch Sitting with soles of your feet placed together, rest your elbows against your knees. Keeping your back straight, try to push your knees down without straining. Hold for 10 seconds and then try to push your knees down a little further and hold for another 10 seconds. Slowly relax.

36 Chest stretch Standing with your feet hip-width apart and your knees slightly bent, draw your shoulders and arms backwards, keeping your arms straight and as high as possible. Hold the extreme position for 10 seconds then slowly relax your arms down to your sides.

37 Shoulder stretch Bring your right arm up over your head and down your back while bringing your left arm up behind your back. Clasp your fingers together if possible and hold the extreme position for 10 seconds. Slowly release then repeat the exercise reversing the position of the arms.

REMOBILISE

Turn back to pages 68-69 and repeat Exercises 1–4. Perform just a few repetitions of each movement to re-mobilise your joints and leave your body feeling great.

VEGETARIAN DIETING

With the increasing interest in vegetarian eating I feel it is important to offer specific guidance to my low-fat dieters. As I am not a vegetarian I decided to call upon the expertise of Roselyne Masselin, who runs her own vegetarian cookery school (La Cuisine Imaginaire) in London.

In this chapter Roselyne explains clearly the various aspects of vegetarianism and, in particular, how to create a nutritious and balanced low-fat vegetarian diet. She also supplies you with a range of practical, easy-to-follow recipes that are low in fat and high in fibre – a great combination for the perfect slimming diet.

You don't need to be vegetarian to enjoy making the recipes in this chapter; I find many people I come across want to eat meat only 2 or 3 times a week. These recipes provide quick, healthy meat alternatives for the meals in between. Some of the recipes (Vegetable Mirepoix in Filo Overcoat, Chickpea Couscous, Duo of Courgettes and Flageolets en Salade) are also suitable for dinner parties. However, I feel I should add an explanatory note regarding the inclusion of oil in some of her recipes.

Anyone who reads this or any of my other books will know that oil, whether animal or vegetable based, is included on the Forbidden List, and this rule *still applies* to anyone who is *not* vegetarian. But it must also be understood that I do not at any time recommend a 'no-fat diet'. Such a diet would be unhealthy. My 'low'-fat diets still incorporate sufficient fat within the

foods that are recommended to supply the nutrients necessary for good health. The fat included in the leanest cuts of meat, in poultry and in fish is a valuable part of our diet. However, vegetarians who follow a low-fat diet and who exclude those foods may be eating too little fat and, with this in mind, Roselyne has included a small amount of vegetable oil in some of her recipes. The amount works out at less than a teaspoonful per person. In this context, therefore, oil *is* allowed within my low-fat diet. However, this does not mean you may add it liberally elsewhere!

WHY IS THE INTEREST IN VEGETARIANISM GROWING?

There are various reasons why this way of eating is now more popular than ever.

Health and Fitness

A vegetarian diet offers the excellent combination of:

- plenty of fresh fruits and vegetables, which boost the fibre content in the diet
- An overall low-fat intake – most ingredients (pulses, grain, fruits, and vegetables) have a low-fat content

Changes in Dietary Habits

The general public is now much more willing to

try unusual and exotic ingredients and this has revolutionised eating patterns, opening our eyes to the possibilities of Chinese, Japanese, Indonesian and other international cuisines being tried, tested and enjoyed.

Concern for Animals and the Environment

In the 1990s many people started a new way of thinking along the lines of: 'I do care about animals, the environment and my future'. Approximately half the people who stop eating meat do so for ethical reasons.

HOW TO BE A HEALTHY VEGETARIAN

A vegetarian diet excludes red and white meat, all fish, poultry and animal fats (but, of course, not dairy products).

The diet is based on 5 major food groups which vegetarians should regularly incorporate into their daily diet.

Grains
Barley: made into flour and flakes
Buckwheat: made into flour
Millet: made into flakes
Oats: made into oatmeal and oatflakes
Rice: made into rice cakes, rice flour and rice flakes
Rye: made into flour and bread
Wheat: made into flour, pasta, couscous, bulgar wheat

Pulses
Aduki beans
Blackeyed beans
Brown lentils
Chickpeas
Mung beans

Peas
Red kidney beans
Red split lentils
Split peas

Nuts and Seeds
Brazil nuts
Cashew nuts
Hazelnuts
Peanuts
Pecan nuts
Pine nuts
Walnuts

Dairy Products
Cheese
Milk
Yogurt

Fruits and Vegetables
Selection of all green, red, yellow and orange vegetables
Selection of all fruits

Don't worry if this sounds daunting: all you need to do is mix and match. A breakfast of muesli (grain and dairy products), a light lunch of peanut butter and salad bap (nut and grain and vegetable), and an evening meal of a bean dish such as Tikka Lentil Bake (pulse and vegetable) is a good example of how this can be achieved.

HOW TO REPLACE MEAT PROTEINS

Four of the five aforementioned food groups are rich in protein – grains, pulses, nuts and seeds and dairy products.

However, these foods are not complete proteins in themselves, and therefore you have to combine them in the following ways (see overleaf):

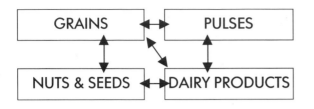

Provided you combine these food groups together in a meal and in the course of the day, you will ensure you receive an adequate protein intake.

Depending on your weight, you should eat between 6–9 oz (150–225g) of 'protein food combinations'; this can easily be achieved by eating a selection of the combinations mentioned above.

New sources of mycoproteins and TVP/TSP (Textured Vegetable Protein/Textured Soya Protein) are available on the market; these products are designed to make the life of the consumer easier as chunks of Quorn or TVP/TSP will absorb the flavour of whatever food they are mixed with and can be added to almost any vegetable-based dish and yield good-quality protein.

B VITAMINS REQUIREMENTS

Requirements of B vitamins vary from one person to another. Factors such as stress, environment, level of activity, etc. affect its levels. To get enough, ensure you eat a diet based on wholefoods; eat wholemeal bread, wholemeal pasta, wholemeal rice and so on as often as possible. As well as boosting your B vitamin levels, these foods will provide extra fibre.

B vitamins are needed for the health of the nervous system and help you cope with everyday pressures. If you feel you are low in B vitamins, sprinkle a little wheatgerm (which should be kept in the fridge) on your cereals and, at the end of the cooking time, on casseroles, as well as on sweets and yogurts, fromage frais, Greek yogurt, and so on.

OTHER VITAMINS, CALCIUM AND IRON

Fruits and vegetables provide an abundance of vitamin C and vitamin A. Dairy products are a good source of calcium. Iron is found in most wholefoods such as pulses – especially lentils – wholegrains, nuts, seeds and dried fruits.

Iron levels can be adversely affected by too much bran. A vegetarian diet should provide enough fibre so there should be no need to sprinkle any bran on your breakfast cereals.

THE INGREDIENTS USED
Grains
Bulgar wheat Made from wheat, bulgar is par-boiled cracked wheat grains. To cook it, all you need to do is pour boiling water over it and let the mixture stand for 15 minutes. (See Mixed Grain and Fresh Coriander Medley, page 85.)

Couscous A derivative of wheat, couscous is made from the same dough as pasta but couscous is shaped into tiny pellets. To cook it, just pour boiling water over and leave to stand for 10 minutes. It will swell up and cook to a light fluffy consistency. (See Chickpea Couscous, page 88.)

Millet An alkaline-forming grain, millet is high in protein. It is cooked in 20 minutes and millet can be substituted for rice in most recipes. (See Three-Layer Millet Bake, page 84.)

Quinoa This is a grain not dissimilar to sesame seeds in appearance. It is cooked in 15 minutes, and its cooked texture is a cross between tapioca and millet. Quinoa has a high protein content and is easily digestible. (See Chickpea Couscous, page 88.)

Risotto rice Often known as arborio, this rice is native of Italy. When cooking, risotto rice swells as it absorbs water and its consistency becomes 'porridgy' and sticky. (See Vegetable Mirepoix in Filo Overcoat, page 82.)

Pulses

Dry varieties All pulses are sold in their dry form as they have a long shelf life this way. They take a long time to prepare as you have to soak them to reconstitute their original shape, and then cook until tender.

Canned varieties Canned pulses, peas and lentils are a very good alternative to the dry ones. Pulses do not lose too much nutritional value when prepared this way. Choose the varieties that have no sugar added.

The Flavourings

Vegetable bouillon powder This is a light vegetable concentrate found in most wholefood shops. It is useful for light casseroles and is also a suitable addition for light soups as this concentrate will not affect its colour.

Vegetable stock cubes Most supermarkets sell their own brands of stock cubes and flavours vary quite a lot; choose the ones with no monosodium glutamate.

Tamari This is a good-quality soya sauce, aged in wood for up to 2 years. A native of Japan, tamari is poorly imitated by Western manufacturers, who try to produce soya sauces within a few weeks and often add monosodium glutamate to strengthen the results. Tamari is found in wholefood shops; if none is available, choose naturally fermented soya sauces.

Marmite Often thought of as containing beef extract, Marmite is actually vegetable-based; it contains the B12 vitamin too. Marmite can help

flavour sauces (use as a gravy alternative) and casseroles.

Ginger juice This is easily made by using unpeeled root ginger. Grate the ginger and squeeze out as much of the juice as possible. (See Tofu Indonesian Style and Stir-Fried Ginger and Sesame Marinade, pages 81 and 85.)

Miscellaneous

Filo pastry This is a very thin pastry which you will find in the frozen food departments in supermarkets. Do not defrost for longer than 2 hours, otherwise it will become very dry and brittle and impossible to work with.

Tofu This is a Japanaese soya bean curd made from the separation of soya curds and whey. Although the process is the same as in cheese-making, tofu has no particular flavour and needs to be cooked with tasty ingredients to improve its appeal.

NOTE

Because of the high-fat content the consumption of nuts and seeds should be restricted whilst following a low-fat diet. It is easy to create complete proteins by combining grains, pulses and dairy products. Roselyne's delicious recipes show you how to do this. However, nuts and seeds need not be completely eliminated as – in the absence of protein foods in the form of meat and poultry – grains, pulses and vegetables are virtually fat-free. These items will make up the bulk of your diet and therefore there is room for some non-animal proteins which do contain some fat. It is, of course, always essential to have sufficient fat in any diet.

When selecting dairy products, always take time to find low-fat brands whenever possible.

VEGETARIAN RECIPES

CHESTNUT PATE

....

(SERVES 4)

1 tablespoon sunflower or
vegetable oil
1 medium turnip, peeled and
diced
4 oz (100g) wholemeal bread
10 oz (250g) tinned whole
chestnuts, drained
2 large eggs
1 tablespoon tamari
2 tablespoons peanut butter
1 level teaspoon garam masala
few drops Tabasco
salt and freshly ground black
pepper

Heat the oil and fry the turnip until golden. Do not overcook.

Meanwhile place the bread in a food processor and process into breadcrumbs. Add the chestnuts and process for a few more seconds until the chestnuts are finely chopped.

Take the mixture out of the food processor, add the eggs and tamari and mix well. Add the cooked turnip, peanut butter, garam masala, Tabasco and seasoning. Stir, making sure that the peanut butter is dissolved.

Line the base of a 1-lb (400g) loaf tin with greaseproof paper; pack the chestnut mix-ture into it and bake in a pre-heated oven at 190°C, 375°F, or Gas Mark 5 for 35–40 minutes. Leave to stand for 10 minutes then turn out. Allow to cool thoroughly before serving.

TIKKA LENTIL BAKE

....

(SERVES 4)

For the base
6 oz (150g) brown lentils
1 tablespoon sunflower or
vegetable oil
6 oz (150g) leeks, cleaned and
chopped
2 cloves garlic, crushed
1 medium carrot, peeled and
diced
4 oz (100g) turnip, peeled and
diced
8 oz (200g) mushrooms, diced
2 tablespoons tomato purée
2–3 tablespoons dark stock (1
teaspoon Marmite in boiling
water)
1 tablespoon tikka paste
2 tablespoons tamari (or other
good quality soya sauce)
salt and freshly ground black
pepper
For the topping
1 lb (400g) potatoes, peeled
and chopped
½ oz (12.5g) butter or
margarine (optional)
4-6 tablespoons semi-
skimmed or skimmed milk

Bring 1 pint (500ml) water to the boil in a saucepan. Add the lentils and boil fast for 10 minutes uncovered. Turn the heat down and simmer until tender, approximately 30 minutes.

Meanwhile heat the oil in a medium saucepan and fry the leeks until soft. Add the garlic, carrot, turnip and mushrooms, and cook, covered, for 10 minutes.

Meanwhile, place the potatoes in a saucepan and bring to the boil. Simmer until tender, then drain and mash with a little butter/margarine and milk.

When the vegetables are tender, add the cooked lentils and tomato purée, stock, tikka paste, tamari/soya sauce and salt and pepper. Bring the mix-ture to the boil and cook to-gether for a few minutes for the flavours to mingle.

Place the lentil mixture in a 2½–3-pint (1.25–1.5 litre) oval ovenproof dish. Top with the mashed potatoes and finish with a decorative pattern, using a fork. You may sprinkle a few sesame seeds on the top and finish with a dot of butter to help with browning.

Bake in a preheated oven at 200°C, 400°F, or Gas Mark 6 for 25 minutes. Serve hot with a selection of steamed vegetables.

If you prefer, you can bake this recipe in individual dishes; cook for 15 minutes.

RICE AND ALMOND PILAFF

(SERVES 4)

6 oz (150g) long grain
wholemeal rice
1 onion, chopped
1 tablespoon sunflower oil
6 oz (150g) green beans,
topped and tailed and halved
across
1 large orange pepper,
chunkily chopped
3½ oz (87.5g) sweetcorn
2 teaspoons bouillon powder
or 1 vegetable stock cube
1 tablespoon creamed
horseradish
salt and freshly ground black
pepper
2 oz (50g) lightly toasted
flaked almonds

Place 12 fl oz (300ml) water in a small saucepan and bring to the boil. Add the rice, bring the mixture back to the boil, turn the heat down, cover with a lid, and simmer for 25 minutes.

Meanwhile fry the onion in the oil until golden brown. Add the green beans and cook for 5 minutes. Add the orange pepper, cover and cook for another few minutes. Add the cooked rice, sweetcorn, bouillon powder (or stock cube), creamed horseradish and seasoning and cook, covered, for a few more minutes. If the mixture seems dry, add a few tablespoons of light stock or water.

Just before serving, stir in the flaked almonds and check the seasoning.

TOFU INDONESIAN STYLE

(SERVES 4)

10 oz (250g) packet regular
tofu
1 tablespoon sunflower oil
4 oz (100g) baby carrots,
peeled and thinly sliced
6 oz (150g) baby sweetcorn,
each stick cut in half at a slant
6 oz (150g) mange tout,
topped and tailed
4 oz (100g) turnip or white
radish, peeled and sliced
For the sauce
2 teaspoons arrowroot
1 tablespoon tamari
1 lime leaf or bay leaf
2 small red and green chillies
2-inch (5cm) piece lemon
grass
2-teaspoons fresh ginger juice
(see note on page 79)

Cube the tofu into 20 pieces and leave it to drain on kitchen paper.

Heat the oil and sweat the vegetables in a semi-covered pan for 5 minutes, stirring from time to time.

Mix all the sauce ingredients together until smooth, add the tofu and pour the sauce and tofu over the vegetables. Replace the lid and cook for 8 minutes.

Season and serve on a bed of cooked rice.

FRESH TAGLIATELLE WITH BLUE CHEESE SAUCE

(SERVES 4)

12 oz (300g) tagliatelle
For the sauce
2 teaspoons arrowroot
½ pint (250ml) semi-skimmed
or skimmed milk
2 oz (50g) blue cheese,
crumbled
salt and freshly ground black
pepper
To garnish
1–2 tablespoons fresh
chopped chives

Cook the tagliatelle as indicated on the packet.

Meanwhile, place the arrowroot in a small saucepan and gradually add the milk, stirring all the time. Then add the blue cheese. Bring the mixture to the boil and simmer for 2 minutes,

81

making sure that the blue cheese is thoroughly melted, then season well.

Serve the sauce on a bed of the tagliatelle and sprinkle the top with the chives.

DUO OF COURGETTES AND FLAGEOLETS EN SALADE

....

(SERVES 4)

12 oz (300g) courgettes, sliced at a slant
½ red onion, sliced
14 oz (350g) tinned flageolet beans, drained and rinsed
salt and freshly ground black pepper
For the dressing
1 tablespoon pesto sauce
2 tablespoons fresh chopped basil
2 tablespoons lemon juice
1 tablespoon olive oil

Steam the courgette slices for 6 minutes. Meanwhile prepare the dressing by mixing all the ingredients together.

When the courgettes are ready, place them in a mixing bowl and pour the dressing on top. Leave to cool and marinate for 10–15 minutes.

Add the onion, flageolet beans and seasoning, mix well but gently. Leave to stand until completely cold.

VEGETABLE MIREPOIX IN FILO OVERCOAT

....

(SERVES 4)

For the pastry
½ packet frozen filo pastry, left to defrost for 2 hours
2 oz (50g) butter, melted
For the mirepoix mixture
3 oz (75g) risotto rice
2 teaspoons bouillon powder or 1 vegetable stock cube
6 fl oz (150ml) water
½ oz (12.5g) butter or margarine
2 shallots or 1 small onion, peeled and chopped
5 oz (125g) baby carrots, peeled and diced finely
8 oz (200g) cauliflower florets, cut into small pieces
4 oz (100g) petits pois
4 oz (100g) fresh spinach, very finely chopped
½ bunch watercress (include some of the stalks)
1 teaspoon fresh chopped thyme
salt and freshly ground black pepper
For the sauce
4 oz (100g) fresh spinach, washed and chopped
½ bunch watercress, chopped
3 fl oz (75ml) semi-skimmed or skimmed milk
2½ fl oz (62.5ml) single cream
½ teaspoon grated lemon rind
salt and freshly ground black pepper

To garnish
a little extra watercress
4 tomatoes

Place the rice with the water and the bouillon powder or stock cube in a small saucepan and bring to the boil; cover and simmer for 20 minutes.

Meanwhile melt the butter or margarine and fry the shallots, carrots and cauliflower until soft. Add the petits pois, spinach and watercress and leave to cook for another few minutes. Add the cooked rice and fresh thyme and season well. Leave to cool.

Unwrap the filo pastry and cut each piece of filo pastry in half, lengthwise. Brush with the melted butter and place some of the filling (about 2 tablespoons) at the end of each leaf. Wrap the filling in the filo pastry, as though a parcel, and brush the top of the pastry with a little extra butter. Place on a lightly greased baking sheet and bake in a preheated oven at 220°C, 425°F, or Gas Mark 7 for 20 minutes or until the pastry is crisp and golden.

Meanwhile make the sauce: place the spinach and watercress in a small saucepan and cook covered on a very low heat for 6–8 minutes with no

Right: Vegetable Mirepoix in Filo Overcoat

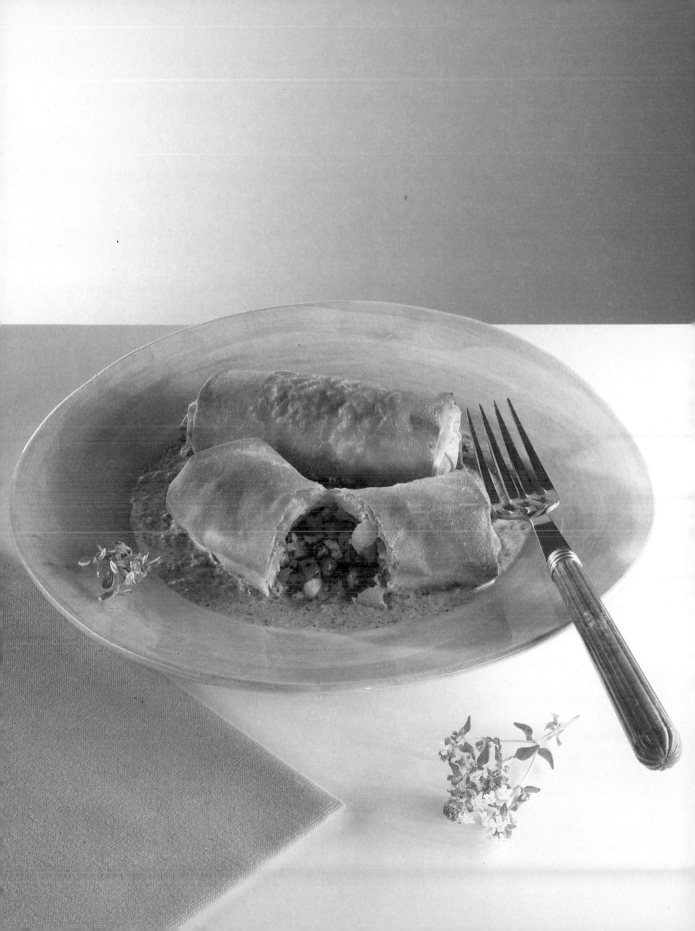

other water than that clinging to the spinach leaves. Add the milk and bring to the boil.

Transfer the mixture into a blender and process until completely smooth. Pour the contents into a clean, small saucepan, add the single cream, lemon rind and seasoning and bring to boiling point.

To serve, pour some of the sauce on to each plate, place the parcels on top and garnish with extra watercress and a tomato rose. Accompany with extra vegetables or a side salad.

QUICK AND LOW-FAT COURGETTE LASAGNE

....

(SERVES 4)

1 tablespoon olive oil
1 onion, peeled and chopped
8 oz (200g) courgettes, diced
1 green pepper, diced finely
14 oz (350g) tinned tomatoes
2 tablespoons tomato purée
2 teaspoons bouillon powder
or 1 vegetable stock cube
2 teaspoons dried basil
salt and freshly ground black
pepper
8 'no pre-cook' wholemeal
lasagne sheets
For the topping
½ pint (250ml) plain natural
yogurt or low-fat fromage frais
1 egg, beaten
1 teaspoon ground cumin

Heat the oil in a frying pan and fry the onion until tender. Add the courgettes and green pepper and fry gently for a few more minutes. Add the tomatoes, tomato purée, bouillon powder (or vegetable stock cube) and dried basil, and bring the mixture to the boil. Break the tomatoes and simmer for 10 minutes. Season well.

Place a layer of the tomato mixture on the base of a lasagne dish, top with 4 sheets of lasagne, then repeat the tomato layer and lasagne sheets; finish with a layer of the tomato mixture.

Whisk the topping ingredients together and pour over.

Bake in a preheated oven at 190°C, 375°F, or Gas Mark 5 for 25–30 minutes.

Serve hot or cold with a crisp salad.

THREE-LAYER MILLET BAKE

....

(SERVES 4)

8 oz (200g) millet
2 teaspoons bouillon powder
or 1½ vegetable stock cubes
For the base
1 tablespoon olive oil
1 onion, peeled and finely
chopped
8 oz (200g) courgettes,
chopped
2 cloves garlic, crushed
14 oz (350g) tinned chopped
tomatoes
1–2 tablespoons tomato purée
1 teaspoon fresh mixed herbs
2 tablespoons fresh chopped
parsley
salt and freshly ground black
pepper
For the topping
½ pint (250ml) plain yogurt
4 oz (100g) strong cheddar
cheese, grated
a good pinch of ground cumin

Place the millet and the bouillon powder or stock cubes in a medium-sized saucepan. Add ¾ pint (375ml) water, bring the mixture to the boil, cover with a lid and simmer for 20 minutes.

Meanwhile make the tomato sauce. Heat the oil and fry the onion, courgettes and garlic on a medium heat until tender. Add the tomatoes and tomato purée and boil for 5 minutes. Add the herbs and seasoning.

Place the yogurt in a mixing bowl and add the grated cheese and cumin.

Place the tomato mixture in a 2½–3 pint (1.25–1.5 litre) ovenproof dish, cover with the cooked millet and finish with the yogurt layer. Bake in a pre-heated oven at 190°C, 375°F, or Gas Mark 5 for 30 minutes or until the yogurt is set.

Leave to stand for 5 minutes and serve hot with salad.

MIXED GRAIN AND FRESH CORIANDER MEDLEY

(SERVES 4)

½ oz (12.5g) butter or vegetable margarine
10 oz (250g) field mushrooms, halved across and sliced
1 rounded teaspoon Marmite
1 tablespoon tamari
4 oz (100g) couscous
4 oz (100g) bulgar wheat
4–6 tablespoons fresh chopped coriander
2 beef tomatoes, sliced
2 oz (50g) grated mozarella cheese
salt and freshly ground black pepper

Heat the butter or margarine and fry the mushrooms on a medium heat until tender.

Make up some stock by mixing Marmite and tamari with ¾ pint (375ml) boiling water. Add the stock to the mushrooms, then add the couscous, bulgar wheat and all but 1 tablespoon fresh chopped coriander. Season well.

Place the mixture in a 2½–3 pint (1.25–1.5 litre) ovenproof dish and top with the sliced tomatoes. Sprinkle the cheese on top of the tomatoes and finish with the remaining fresh coriander. Season with plenty of black pepper and a little salt.

Bake in a pre-heated oven at 200°C, 400°F, or Gas Mark 6 for 20 minutes. Leave to stand for 5 minutes prior to serving.

STIR-FRIED VEGETABLES WITH GINGER AND SESAME MARINADE

(SERVES 4)

1½ tablespoons sunflower oil
1 onion, cut in half and shredded
12 oz (300g) mange tout, topped and tailed
1 large red pepper, cut into strips
10 oz (250g) mung beansprouts
1 medium Chinese cabbage, shredded
For the marinade
3 tablespoons fresh ginger juice (see page 79)
3 teaspoons arrowroot
3 tablespoons tamari
1 teaspoon toasted sesame oil
3 fl oz (75ml) light stock or water

Heat the oil in a wok and quickly fry the onion until soft. Add the mange tout and cook for about 1 minute, stirring all the time to stop them from going brown. Add the red pepper and cook for another 3 minutes. Add the beansprouts and Chinese cabbage and cook until both look tender, stirring from time to time.

Meanwhile make the marinade by mixing all the ingredients together thoroughly. Add the marinade to the vegetables and bring the mixture back to the boil. Cover with a lid, turn the heat down and cook for a further 3–4 minutes to finish cooking the vegetables.

Serve straight away on a bed of cooked rice.

BROCCOLI GRATINE WITH CHEESE AND CANNELLINI TOPPING

....

(SERVES 4)

For the base
1 lb (400g) broccoli florets
6 oz (150g) carrots, peeled and sliced
For the topping
14 oz (350g) tinned cannellini beans, drained and rinsed
7 fl oz (175ml) semi-skimmed or skimmed milk
salt and freshly ground black pepper
2–3 oz (50–75g) cheddar cheese, grated
To garnish
a few flaked almonds (optional)

Steam the broccoli and carrots together until *al dente*.

Meanwhile make the topping: blend the beans and milk together until smooth, transfer the mixture into a saucepan, bring to the boil and simmer for 2–3 minutes. Season well

and leave to cool.

Place the broccoli and carrots in a 2½–3-pint (1.25–1.5 litre) ovenproof dish; pour the cannellini mixture over and top with the cheese. Sprinkle the almonds on top (if used).

Bake in a preheated oven at 200°C, 400°F, or Gas Mark 6 for 15 minutes or until golden. Serve hot.

CREAMY HORSERADISH AND WATERCRESS CRUMBLE

....

(SERVES 4)

For the base
6 oz (150g) cauliflower, cut in small florets
4 oz (100g) broccoli florets
8 oz (200g) courgettes, chopped
1 red pepper, diced
2 oz (50g) frozen garden peas
1 medium leek, peeled and chopped
1 oz (25g) butter or margarine
1 oz (25g) wholewheat plain flour
½ pint (250ml) semi-skimmed milk
2 teaspoons creamed horseradish
½ bunch watercress, finely chopped
salt and freshly ground black pepper

For the topping
2 oz (50g) wheat flakes, oat flakes or barley flakes
2 oz (50g) wholewheat breadcrumbs
2 oz (50g) butter or margarine
2 oz (50g) grated cheddar cheese
To garnish
about ½ oz (12.5g) sunflower seeds

Steam the cauliflower and broccoli florets for 3 minutes. Add the courgettes and steam for another 2 minutes. Add the red pepper and peas and steam for another 2 minutes. Add the leek and steam for another 2 minutes.

Meanwhile make the sauce. Melt the butter or margarine in a small saucepan and stir in the flour; cook the roux for 2 minutes. Take the pan off the heat and gradually add the milk, stirring all the time. Put the pan back on the heat and bring to the boil, stirring all the time. Turn the heat down and simmer for 3 minutes, still stirring. Take the pan off the heat again and stir in the horseradish, watercress and seasoning. Finally, fold in the steamed vegetables carefully.

Place the mixture in a 3-pint

Right: Broccoli Gratiné with Cheese and Cannellini Topping

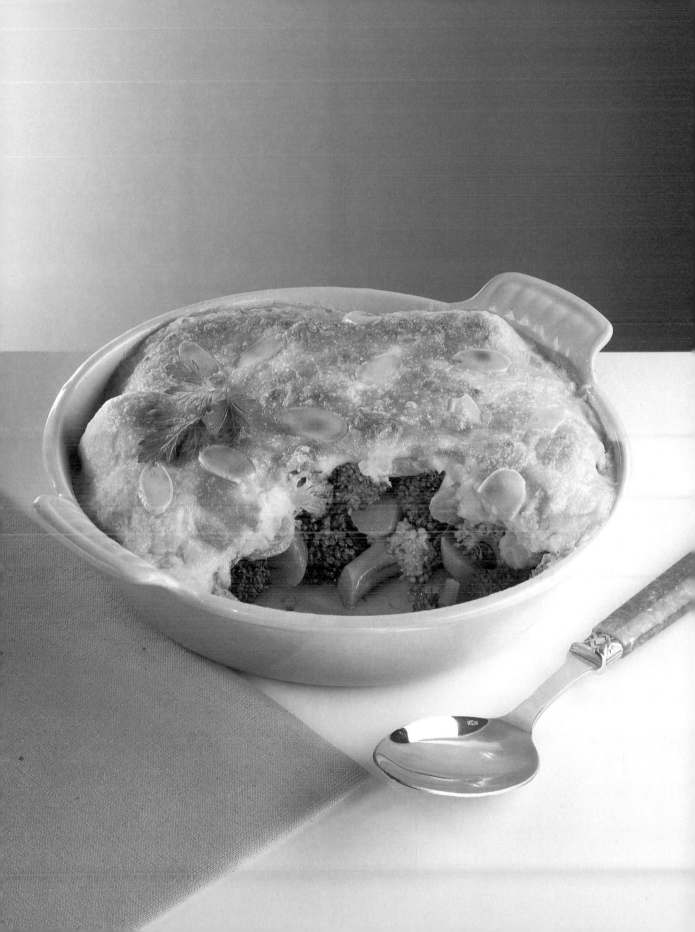

(1.5 litre) ovenproof dish.

Mix the flakes and bread-crumbs together. Rub the butter or margarine into the mixture and add the grated cheese.

Cover the vegetable mixture with the crumble topping and bake in a preheated oven at 190°C, 375°F, or Gas Mark 5 for 25 minutes or until crisp and golden on top.

Serve hot with crisp salad.

TRICOLOUR PASTA RISOTTO

....

(SERVES 3–4 PEOPLE)

1 tablespoon olive oil
1 onion, cut in half and shredded
8 oz (200g) courgettes, thinly cut lengthwise – discard the first slice, then cut in 1½ inch (3.7mm) long pieces across
1 red pepper, cut into 1½ inch (3.7mm) long strips
3 oz (75g) petits pois
8 oz (200g) tricolour pasta spirals
¾ pint (375ml) water
1 vegetable stock cube
14 oz (350g) tinned tomatoes
2 teaspoons freshly chopped or 1 teaspoon dry marjoram
salt and freshly ground black pepper
To serve
2 oz (50g) strong cheese, grated

Heat the olive oil and fry the onion and courgettes for 3 minutes. Add the red pepper, peas, pasta, water and stock cube, tomatoes and marjoram. Bring back to the boil, cover, and simmer for 20 minutes.

Season, then leave the mixture to stand for 5 minutes before serving with grated cheese and a crisp salad.

CHICKPEA COUSCOUS

....

(SERVES 4)

1 tablespoon sunflower or vegetable oil
2 medium carrots, peeled and halved lengthwise and sliced across
1 medium to large potato, peeled and chopped
½ cauliflower, cut into florets
8 oz (200g) courgettes, chunkily chopped
2–3 oz (50–75g) green beans, cut in half across
1 teaspoon ground coriander
2 vegetable stock cubes
¾ pint (375ml) water or light stock
¼ pint (125ml) ready-made tomato sauce
1 medium red pepper, diced
4 oz (100g) okra, topped and tailed and cut in half across
2 green chillies
1 tablespoon tikka paste or other marinating paste

14 oz (350g) tinned chickpeas, drained and rinsed
salt and freshly ground black pepper

Heat the oil in a medium-sized saucepan and gently fry the carrots, potato and cauliflower. Stir the mixture from time to time to prevent it sticking to the bottom of the pan. Add the courgettes, green beans and coriander and cook slowly for another 5 minutes.

Add the stock cubes, water or stock, tomato sauce, red pepper, okra, chillies, tikka paste and chickpeas and cook for 20–30 minutes.

Season well and serve hot on a bed of cooked couscous, quinoa or rice.

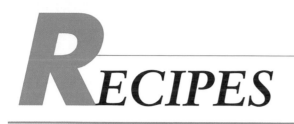

RECIPES

In this section all recipes included in the 28-day programme appear under the following headings:

Breakfasts

Lunches

Dinners

Starters and Soups

Main Courses: meat

Main Courses: poultry and game

Main Courses: fish

Main Courses: vegetarian (see also pages 80-88)

Side Dishes: salads and vegetables

Desserts

Dressings

For further breakfast, lunch and dinner suggestions, please refer back to the daily diet plans.

Ideas for healthy packed lunches for children can be found on pages 151-154 and Christmas recipes on pages 159-170.

For convenience, the following conversion rates have been used throughout this recipe section:

1 oz = 25g
1 fl oz = 25ml
½ pint = 250ml

BREAKFASTS

BANANA MILK SHAKE

(SERVES 1)

1 medium banana
4 fl oz (100ml) skimmed milk
(in addition to allowance)
5 oz (125g) diet yogurt, any
flavour

Place all the ingredients in a food processor and liquidise. Serve in a tall glass.

HOME-MADE MUESLI

(SERVES 1)

1 eating apple
½ oz (12.5g) oats
½ oz (12.5g) sultanas or half
banana
2 teaspoons bran
milk from allowance or 3 oz
(75g) natural yogurt
honey (optional)

Grate or chop the apple. Mix all the ingredients together and add honey to taste if required.

Alternatively, mix all the ingredients (except the banana) together the night before and leave to soak overnight in skimmed milk.

PINEAPPLE BOAT

....

(SERVES 2)

1 medium-sized fresh
pineapple
8 oz (200g) seasonal fruit of
your choice
10 oz (250g) diet yogurt, any
flavour
2 cherries or strawberries, to
decorate

Divide the pineapple into 2
halves from top to bottom. Do
not cut away the leaves – they
add to the decorative look. Cut
away flesh with a grapefruit
knife and cut this flesh into
cubes, removing hard core.

Prepare other fruit – wash
and cut into bite-sized pieces
and mix with pineapple. Pile
into hollowed-out pineapple
halves and dress with yogurt.

Serve chilled and decorated
with a cherry or strawberry.

PORRIDGE

....

(SERVES 1)

1 oz (25g) porridge oats
½ pint (250ml) cold water
1 oz (25g) sultanas
liquid sweetener
1 teaspoon liquid honey

Place the porridge oats and the
water in a small milk saucepan
and heat gently until boiling.
Add the sultanas and leave to
simmer for 5 minutes. Add the
liquid sweetener. Leave
covered overnight.

Stir well and reheat until
thoroughly hot.

To serve, pour milk from
your allowance into a cereal
dish, tip the porridge into this
and it will float. Now pour on
the liquid honey.

LUNCHES

....

CHEESE, PRAWN AND ASPARAGUS SALAD

....

(SERVES 2)

4 oz (100g) low-fat cottage
cheese
6 oz (150g) peeled prawns
4 tablespoons chopped and
diced cucumber
freshly ground black pepper
lettuce or watercress
8 oz
(200g) canned asparagus
tips

Mix the cottage cheese, prawns
and cucumber together. Season
with pepper to taste.

Lay the mixture on a bed of
shredded lettuce or watercress
and decorate with the asparagus tips.

CHEESE AND APRICOT PEARS

....

(SERVES 4)

4 ripe pears
lemon juice
8 oz (200g) low-fat cottage
cheese
4 tablespoons apricot jam or
preserve

Peel the pears, cut in half
lengthways and remove the
core. Brush with lemon juice to

prevent discoloration.

Fill with cottage cheese mixed with apricot jam or preserve.

Serve chilled.

CHEESY STUFFED POTATOES

....

(SERVES 1)

1 medium-sized potato, baked in its jacket
2 oz (50g) low-fat cottage cheese
1 oz (25g) low-fat cheddar cheese
1 teaspoon French mustard
3 tablespoons skimmed milk
freshly ground black pepper and salt to taste
paprika

Preheat oven to 190°C, 375°F, Gas Mark 5. Cut the pre-cooked potato in half lengthways and carefully scoop out the pulp with a spoon, leaving a ¼-inch (0.6 cm) shell.

Place the potato pulp in a large bowl. Add remaining ingredients except the paprika. Mash with a fork or potato masher until mixture is well blended. Spoon the mixture into the empty potato shells. Sprinkle with paprika and bake in a preheated oven for 30 minutes.

CHICKEN LIVER SALAD

....

(SERVES 2)

6 spring onions
2 tomatoes
2 inches (5 cm) cucumber
2 rashers back bacon
4 oz (100g) chicken or duck livers
freshly ground black pepper
½ slice (½ oz/12.5g) bread
Dressing
1 teaspoon French mustard
3 tablespoons lemon juice
1 tablespoon orange juice
1 tablespoon wine vinegar
salt and black pepper

Prepare the oil-free dressing by placing all the ingredients in a jar and shaking well.

Prepare the salad by chopping the spring onions and dry-frying them in a non-stick pan. Quarter the tomatoes and finely chop the cucumber. Mix together, pour the dressing over and toss well.

Trim all the fat from the bacon, grill well and chop into small pieces. Wash and trim the livers and dry-fry with black pepper in a non-stick pan. Toast the bread and cut into tiny squares.

Arrange the salad in 2 bowls and just before serving add the bacon, livers and toast squares to the centre of each bowl. Serve immediately.

CHILLI BACON POTATOES

....

(SERVES 1)

2 oz (50g) lean bacon
1 small onion
4 mushrooms
2 tablespoons chilli sauce
1 medium-sized baked potato

Chop the bacon into small pieces. Peel the onion and chop finely. Wash and trim the mushrooms and chop.

Dry-fry the bacon, onion and mushrooms in a non-stick frying pan until cooked. Add the chilli sauce, mix well and keep warm.

Remove cooked potato from the oven or microwave, slice in half lengthways, top with the chilli bacon mixture and serve.

CHILLI SALAD

....

(SERVES 4)

1 lb (400g) potatoes
1 green pepper
1 red pepper
4 spring onions
2 oz (50g) mushrooms
7½ oz (187.5g) tinned kidney beans
few drops Tabasco sauce
¼ teaspoon chilli powder
5 tablespoons natural yogurt

Peel and dice the potatoes and boil for 15–20 minutes until cooked. Allow to cool. Deseed and dice both peppers. Slice the spring onions thinly. Wash, trim and slice the mushrooms. Drain the tinned kidney beans and rinse well under running water.

Mix the cooked potato, all the fresh vegetables and kidney beans together in a large bowl. Keep chilled.

In a separate bowl, mix together the Tabasco sauce, chilli powder and yogurt, and pour over the prepared salad. Combine thoroughly and serve.

CHINESE APPLE SALAD

....

(SERVES 2–4)

1 red apple
1 green apple
few radishes
2 sticks celery
spring onions
curly lettuce to decorate
1 tablespoon lemon juice
6 oz (150g) fresh beansprouts
Sweet 'n' Sour dressing
1½ tablespoons lemon juice
1 level tablespoon clear honey
few drops soy sauce

Slice both apples, the radishes, celery and spring onions.

In a large salad bowl, mix the apples and lemon juice thoroughly, then add the beansprouts, radishes, celery and spring onions. Decorate the edges of the bowl with curly lettuce.

Shake all the dressing ingredients together in a screw-top jar and pour over the salad.

Toss well and serve immediately.

CLUB SANDWICH

....

(SERVES 1)

2 oz (50g) uncooked lean bacon
3 slices bread
1 teaspoon reduced-oil salad dressing (any brand)
1 teaspoon tomato ketchup
½ teaspoon mustard
1 oz (25g) cooked chicken
1 tomato
shredded lettuce leaves
4 cocktail sticks

Grill the bacon until well cooked and crisp. Toast the bread and spread one slice with reduced-oil salad dressing, the second slice with tomato ketchup, and the third with mustard. Slice the chicken and tomato and place on the first slice. Next, add the toast spread with ketchup, then add the bacon followed by shredded lettuce. Top with the remaining piece of toast (spread with mustard).

Press together firmly. Cut into 4 triangles crossways and pierce each quarter-segment with a cocktail stick to hold it together. To serve, arrange each sandwich quarter on its long edge and serve immediately.

COURGETTE AND TOMATO SALAD

....

(SERVES 4)

2 small heads chicory
4 tomatoes
2 courgettes
1 bunch radishes
5 oz (125 g) low-fat fromage frais or yogurt
½ teaspoon French mustard
1 tablespoon chopped gherkins or 1 tablespoon chopped spring onions
1 tablespoon chopped parsley
salt and pepper

Wash the chicory. Reserve a few leaves for garnishing and slice the rest. Skin and seed the tomatoes and chop the flesh coarsely. Trim the courgettes, cut into 2–3 pieces and slice lengthways, then cut into matchstick-sized pieces. Coarsely grate half the radishes and slice the rest.

Right: Chicken Liver Salad

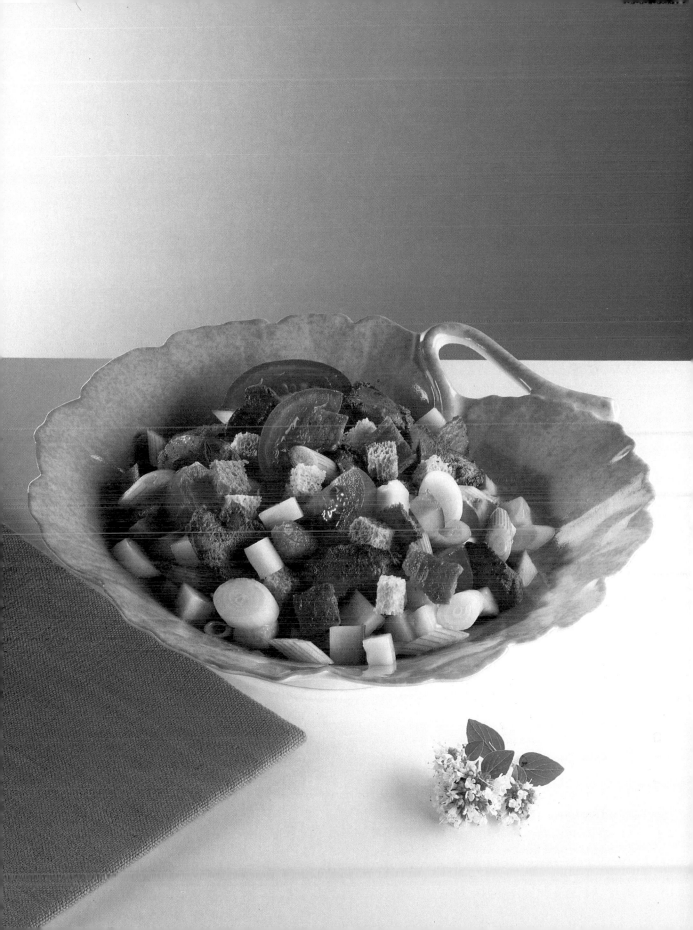

Mix together the fromage frais or yogurt, French mustard, the gherkins or spring onions, and chopped parsley. Season to taste.

Mix the sliced chicory, tomatoes, courgettes and grated radishes together. Fold in the sauce and pile the salad on to a dish. Garnish each end of the dish with the reserved leaves of chicory. Arrange the sliced radishes down the side of the dish. Chill until required.

CUCUMBER BOATS WITH TUNA

....

(SERVES 4)

This dish is suitable for an hors-d'oeuvre for a dinner party or for a cold lunch, served with additional salad vegetables. It can also be made with tinned salmon.

1 cucumber
2 whites of hard-boiled eggs
8 oz (200g) tinned tuna in brine
4 oz (100g) Quark or other low-fat soft cheese or cottage cheese
1 teaspoon made-up mustard
1 tablespoon lemon juice
1 tablespoon chopped parsley
1 tablespoon chopped chives or spring onions
salt and pepper
a few lettuce leaves

Peel the cucumber, cut off the ends and cut in half. Then slice each half in two lengthways. Remove the seeds with a ball-cutter or teaspoon and discard. Blanch the cucumber shells in boiling salted water for 3–5 minutes. Drain and chill under cold running water. Drain well again, then dry on kitchen paper.

Chop the egg whites and keep to one side.

Drain the tuna fish and, using a fork, mash together with the Quark, low-fat cheese or cottage cheese and the mustard and lemon juice. If you prefer a smoother mixture, purée the fish and other ingredients in a food processor or liquidiser. Stir in most of the parsley, and chives or spring onions, and season to taste.

Fill the cucumber shells with the mixture and arrange on lettuce-covered dish or individual plates. Sprinkle the chopped egg whites and remaining herbs over the top. Chill in the refrigerator until required.

CURRIED CHICKEN AND YOGURT SALAD

....

(SERVES 1)

3 oz (75g) cooked chicken breast
5 oz (125g) low-fat natural yogurt
1 teaspoon curry powder
unlimited green salad vegetables

Cube the chicken breast. Mix yogurt and curry powder together and stir in the chicken.

Serve on a bed of fresh green salad vegetables.

KIWIFRUIT AND HAM OPEN SANDWICH

....

(SERVES 1)

1 kiwifruit
1 tablespoon reduced-oil salad dressing (any brand)
1 oz (25g) lean ham
2 oz (50g) French loaf
black pepper (optional)

Cut the loaf lengthways. Spread the dressing on to the bread, shred the ham and place on top of the bread. Garnish with peeled and sliced kiwifruit.

Add black pepper if desired.

KIWIFRUIT MOUSSE

(SERVES 2)

This unusual and tempting dish features kiwifruit filled with paprika cheese in a sweet sharp dressing. For a hot summer's day this tasty, cool and refreshing lunch is hard to beat.

4 kiwifruit
2 oz (50g) low-fat soft cheese
½ level teaspoon paprika
freshly ground black pepper
1 tablespoon lemon juice
1 teaspoon white wine vinegar
salt

Remove both ends of each kiwifruit with a sharp knife. Do not peel. Using an apple corer, carefully remove the centre of each fruit. Reserve. Mix together the cheese, paprika, and black pepper to taste. Fill the hollowed centres of the kiwifruit with the cheese mixture. Chill.

Chop the reserved fruit cores finely, and add the lemon juice and white wine vinegar. Mix this kiwifruit dressing well with a fork, and season to taste.

Peel the filled kiwifruit carefully. Cut each into 4 thick slices. Arrange on plates over evenly distributed kiwifruit dressing. Serve chilled.

OAT AND CHEESE LOAF

(SERVES 4)

8 oz (200g) porridge oats
1 large onion
1 clove garlic
¼ teaspoon sage
¼ teaspoon thyme
¼ teaspoon ground mixed spice
salt and pepper to taste
8 oz (200g) low-fat cottage cheese
4 egg whites

Very lightly oil a 4 × 8 inch (10 × 20 cm) baking tin or spray with a non-stick cooking spray. Combine all the dry ingredients in a large bowl and mix well. In another bowl, combine the cottage cheese and egg whites and beat with a fork or wire whisk until blended. Add to the dry mixture, mixing until all the ingredients are moistened.

Press the mixture firmly into the prepared baking tin, cover with tin foil, and bake in a preheated oven at 180°C, 350°F, or Gas Mark 4 for 25 minutes. Remove the foil and continue baking for a further 25 minutes. Allow to stand for 5 minutes before turning on to a serving plate. Serve with unlimited vegetables or salad.

ORIENTAL STIR-FRY

(SERVES 4)

12 oz (300g) potatoes
1 large red pepper
6 oz (150g) mushrooms
6 oz (150g) frozen sweetcorn
6 oz (150g) cauliflower florets
6 oz (150g) beansprouts
3 tablespoons soy sauce
3 tablespoons Worcestershire sauce
4 tablespoons Parmesan cheese

Peel and grate the potatoes and rinse well. Dry fry them in a non-stick frying pan for 2 minutes.

Deseed the pepper and dice. Wash, trim and slice the mushrooms. Add sweetcorn, diced pepper and cauliflower florets and fry for 5 minutes. Add remaining ingredients and fry for a further 2 minutes.

Serve immediately with 1 tablespoon grated Parmesan cheese sprinkled over each serving.

PRAWN AND PASTA SALAD

....

(SERVES 4)

1 lb (400g) cooked medium-sized pasta shells
1 lb (400g) prawns, peeled, deveined, and cooked
5 oz (125g) natural yogurt
1 tablespoon tomato purée
few drops Tabasco sauce to taste
3 spring onions

Combine the pasta shells and prawns in a serving bowl.

In a small bowl, stir together the yogurt, tomato purée and Tabasco sauce. Pour on to the pasta mixture and toss well.

Sprinkle with finely chopped spring onions just before serving at room temperature or very slightly chilled.

Serve with a green salad.

RICE SALAD

....

(SERVES 1)

1 oz (25g) sweetcorn
1 oz (25g) peas
1 green pepper
1 tomato
2-inch (5cm) piece cucumber
4 oz (100g) [cooked weight] cold cooked brown rice
soy sauce
black pepper and pinch of salt

Cook the sweetcorn and peas in the same pan and allow to cool. Meanwhile, prepare the vegetables. Deseed the green pepper and tomato. Chop all vegetables very finely and mix with the rice, sweetcorn and peas. Add soy sauce and seasoning to taste. Serve cold.

SALAD SURPRISE

....

(SERVES 1)

4 oz (100g) low-fat cottage cheese
1 tablespoon reduced-oil salad dressing (any brand)
1 oz (25g) sweetcorn, cooked
unlimited tomatoes, cucumber, spring onions and green pepper, all finely chopped
salt and black pepper
4 Ryvitas

Mix the cottage cheese with the reduced-oil salad dressing. Add the sweetcorn and finely chopped vegetables. Mix well and season to taste.

Serve with the Ryvitas.

SAVOURY FRENCH BREAD RINGS

....

(SERVES 3–4)

1 small French loaf
8 oz (200g) tinned tuna or salmon in brine
6–8 oz (150–200g) Quark or low-fat soft cheese
1 tablespoon chopped chives or spring onions
1–2 teaspoons chopped capers (optional)
2 tablespoons lemon juice
salt and black pepper
1 small lettuce
4 tomatoes

Cut the French loaf in half lengthways and scrape out some of the bread from both pieces to make a semicircle hollow in each. (Use the scraped-out bread to make breadcrumbs in other recipes.)

Drain the tuna or salmon and place it in a bowl with the Quark or other low-fat soft cheese. Mix well together and stir in the chives or spring onions and capers (if used). Season to taste with lemon juice, salt and black pepper.

Pile the tuna mixture down the length of one piece of bread. Cover with the other piece. Wrap the bread in aluminium foil and roll the parcel lightly so that the mixture evenly fills the centre of the bread. Refrigerate until ready to serve.

To serve, cut the bread in ½–1-inch (1.25–2.5cm) slices and serve with the lettuce and tomatoes. This is ideal for a picnic lunch.

SMOKED MACKEREL PATE

. . . .

(SERVES 3–4)

4 oz (100g) smoked mackerel
8 oz (200g) low-fat cottage cheese
1–2 teaspoons horseradish sauce
2 teaspoons lemon juice
salt and white pepper

Skin the mackerel and remove any bones. Break into medium-sized pieces.

Place all the ingredients in a food processor or liquidiser. If using a liquidiser, it may be advisable to purée the mixture in 2–3 batches. Purée until smooth.

Taste and add more horse-radish sauce, lemon juice, salt or pepper if desired.

Turn out into a dish, cover and chill well until required.

Serves 3–4 with a salad, or in 2 oz (50g) bread rolls with salad, for lunch. Will serve 6 as an hors-d'oeuvre with 1 oz toast per person.

SPRING SALAD

. . . .

(SERVES 1)

Unlimited amount of shredded lettuce, chopped cucumber and any other green salad
1 apple
1 kiwifruit
1 orange
1 pear
2 oz (50g) cooked cold chicken or prawns

Place lettuce and green salad on a large dinner plate. Lay slices of the various fruits around the edge of the plate. In the centre, place chopped chicken or prawns.

Serve with a Marie Rose or Garlic Dressing (see recipes, page 146).

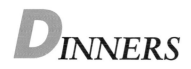

DINNERS

STARTERS AND SOUPS

CRUDITES

. . . .

(SERVES 4)

Cut or break sticks or sprigs of raw cucumber, carrots, celery, green and red peppers and cauliflower and arrange in separate piles around a large serving dish. In the centre of the dish place a small pot of Garlic or Mint Yogurt Dip (see recipe) or any low-fat dip of your choice.

CHESTNUT PATE

. . . .

(See page 80)

GARLIC OR MINT YOGURT DIP

. . . .

5 oz (125g) low-fat natural yogurt
1 clove garlic, finely chopped, or 2 sprigs fresh mint, finely chopped
4 oz (100g) cottage cheese

Mix the yogurt, garlic or mint, and cottage cheese together. Serve in a small dish, accompanied by Crudités (see recipe, page 97).

CRUNCHY VEGETABLE DIP

....

This dip can be served with unlimited quantities of crunchy vegetables and fruits.

carrots
celery
cucumber
cauliflower
apples
2 tablespoons reduced-oil salad dressing
4 oz (100g) cottage cheese

Cut the vegetables and apples into 2-inch (5cm) sticks. Mix together the reduced-oil dressing and the cottage cheese.

To serve, arrange the vegetables attractively on a plate and place the dip in a small bowl.

MELON AND PRAWN SALAD

....

(SERVES 2)

1 melon
4 oz (100g) prawns

Halve the melon and remove seeds. Scoop out flesh of melon with a ball-scoop. Mix the melon balls carefully with the shelled prawns, and replace in empty melon shells. Serve chilled.

MELON WITH STRAWBERRIES

....

(SERVES 4)

2 ogen or honeydew melons
8 oz (200g) strawberries, hulled and washed

Cut the melons in half and remove all the seeds. Trim off a tiny slice of the skin at the base of each half so that they will sit securely on the dish. Fill each half with sliced strawberries.

The melons will look even better if you follow the Vandyke method when cutting them in half, by cutting jagged V's into the side of the melon.

MELON WITH GINGER

....

(SERVES 4)

2 melons, halved, or 1 large honeydew melon, cut into quarters
ground ginger

Remove all seeds from the melon(s). Chill and serve with ground ginger to taste.

MINTY MELON AND YOGURT SALAD

....

(SERVES 4)

1 melon
1 stem mint
10 oz (250g) low-fat natural yogurt
caster sugar to taste

Cut the melon in half and scoop out the seeds. Remove as many melon balls as possible with a ball-cutter or peel the melon and cut the flesh into dice.

Wash and dry the mint. Reserve a few small sprigs for garnishing and chop the rest. Mix the yogurt and mint together and add sugar to taste.

Mix the melon with the yogurt and mint. Cover and refrigerate until required.

To serve, pile into individual dishes and garnish with the reserved sprigs of mint.

RATATOUILLE

....

(See page 135)

SMOKED MACKEREL PATE

....

(See page 97)

SPICY MUSHROOMS

....

(SERVES 4)

1 lb (800g) mushrooms
1 tablespoon lemon juice
1 teaspoon fresh chopped
parsley
1 teaspoon fresh chopped
chives
2 cloves garlic
1 small onion
salt and freshly ground black
pepper
2 chicken stock cubes
7 fl oz (175ml) hot water

Wash and trim the mush-rooms, leaving the stalks in place to prevent shrinkage. Place the mushrooms in an ovenproof dish with the stalks upwards. Sprinkle with lemon juice, parsley, chives, crushed garlic and peeled and grated onion. Season well with the salt and pepper.

Dissolve the stock cubes in the hot water and pour around the mushrooms.

Bake for about 20 minutes in a moderate oven at 180°C, 350°F, or Gas Mark 4. Serve immediately in preheated small dishes.

TUNA PATE WITH CRUDITES

....

(SERVES 4)

8 oz (200g) canned tuna in
brine
3 oz (75g) low-fat natural
yogurt
2 tablespoons reduced-oil
salad dressing (any brand)
1 teaspoon lemon juice
1 teaspoon chopped fresh
parsley
small sticks or sprigs of any of
the following: cucumber,
carrots, celery, red and green
peppers, cauliflower

Drain the tuna and remove any skin or bones. Place tuna in bowl and mash with a fork. Add the yogurt, reduced-oil salad dressing and lemon juice and mix well. Place into 4 small ramekin dishes, pressing down the pâté with the back of a spoon. Refrigerate for at least 2 hours before serving.

Sprinkle the pâté with freshly chopped parsley just before serving and serve with the crudités, arranged attractively on a plate.

WALDORF SALAD

....

(SERVES 4)

1 head of celery
2 apples
6 oz (150g) canned water
chestnuts
2 tablespoons lemon juice
2 oz (50g) sultanas
5 oz (125g) low-fat natural
yogurt
3 tablespoons reduced-oil
salad dressing (any brand)
salt and pepper to taste

Core and chop the apples. Wash and chop the celery and water chestnuts and mix together with the lemon juice and apples.

Mix together all other ingredients in a bowl and pour over salad. Stir well to ensure a thorough coating. Keep chilled until ready to serve.

Serve on a bed of lettuce within two hours of preparation.

BEEF AND VEGETABLE SOUP

....

(SERVES 4)

8 oz (200g) onions
2 large beef bones bought
from a butcher
1 teaspoon mixed herbs
4 oz (100g) potatoes
8 oz (200g) carrots
15 oz (375g) canned peas
3 beef stock cubes
salt and freshly ground black
pepper

For best results, prepare the beef stock a day in advance. To make the stock, peel and chop the onions and place them together with the bones and the mixed herbs in a large saucepan with enough water to cover them. Cover with a lid and boil for 1–2 hours. Remove the bones and allow the stock to cool, then place it in the refrigerator. When the stock is thoroughly chilled, skim off any fat that has solidified on the top. Return to the refrigerator and leave overnight. The stock is now ready for the preparation of the soup.

Peel and chop the potatoes and carrots and place these with the peas and the beef stock in a large saucepan. Bring to the boil, add the stock cubes and simmer for 30 minutes. Season, and serve hot.

CHICKEN AND MUSHROOM SOUP

....

(SERVES 4)

1 onion
1 carrot
bones of one chicken
2 pints (1 litre) vegetable stock
1 chicken stock cube
1 teaspoon mixed herbs
sprinkling of garlic salt, if
desired
black pepper to taste
1 bay leaf
6 peppercorns
4 oz (100g) mushrooms

Peel and slice the onion, slice the carrot and place all ingredients except mushrooms in a large saucepan and cover. Bring to the boil and simmer for approximately 2–3 hours. Taste. If too weak, boil a little faster and remove the saucepan lid until liquid has reduced and it tastes appetising. Strain away bones and vegetables and pour the soup back into the saucepan.

Wash and slice the mushrooms and add to the soup. Cover and cook for 10 minutes.

Serve piping hot.

CHICKEN SOUP

....

(SERVES 4)

1 chicken carcass or 3 chicken
stock cubes
2 pints (1 litre) vegetable stock
1 teaspoon mixed herbs
1 large onion, peeled and
chopped
2 bay leaves
6 peppercorns
salt and freshly ground black
pepper

Place the chicken carcass or stock cubes in a large saucepan with the vegetable stock and all remaining ingredients. Bring to the boil, cover the pan and simmer for 1–1½ hours. Taste for flavouring and add 1 (additional) stock cube if necessary. Strain the soup through a colander to remove all bones, bay leaves and peppercorns.

Store in a refrigerator when cool and use within 2 days. Reheat to serve.

CHILLED GREEN PEA SOUP

....

(SERVES 4–6)

This recipe is ideal as an hors-d'oeuvre for a summer celebration meal.

*1 lb (400g) young fresh peas
(including the pods) or frozen
peas
1 onion
½ lettuce or 6 large leaves
1 sprig mint
1¼ pints (625ml) chicken
stock
1 teaspoon caster sugar
salt and white pepper
a little extra chicken stock
3 tablespoons low-fat natural
yogurt
1 tablespoon chopped parsley
or chives*

Top and tail the fresh pea pods. (There is no need to shell the peas first.) Wash well and cut each pod into 2 or 3 pieces. Peel and finely chop the onion. Wash and shred the lettuce.

Place the fresh or frozen peas in a large pan with the onion, lettuce, mint, stock and sugar. Season lightly with salt and white pepper. Bring to the boil and simmer for about 30 minutes until the vegetables are tender.

Remove the sprig of mint and purée the soup in a food processor or liquidiser. Rub the soup through a sieve to remove any pieces of skin or pod. Add extra stock if necessary to give the consistency of thin cream. Cool slightly then stir in 2 tablespoons yogurt. Adjust the seasoning if necessary.

Chill well and serve in individual bowls with a teaspoon of yogurt swirled on the top of each. Sprinkle a little chopped parsley or chives over.

CREAMY VEGETABLE SOUP

....

(SERVES 4)

*1¼ lbs (500g) potatoes
8 oz (200g) carrots
2 leeks
2 sticks celery
2½ pints (1.5 litres) vegetable
stock
salt and pepper
2 oz (50g) skimmed milk
powder
1 oz (25g) cornflour*
To garnish
chopped parsley

Peel and dice the potatoes. Dice the carrots and finely chop the leeks and celery. Place all the vegetables in a saucepan with stock. Season, cover and simmer for 20–30 minutes.

Blend the skimmed milk powder and cornflour with a little cold water and stir into the soup. Bring to the boil and simmer for 5 minutes, stirring all the time.

Garnish with chopped parsley.

DUCK SOUP

....

(SERVES 4)

*1 large onion
1 clove garlic
1 duck carcass
2 pints (1 litre) vegetable stock
1 chicken stock cube
1 teaspoon mixed herbs
2 bay leves
6 peppercorns
salt and freshly ground black
pepper*

Peel the onion and chop finely. Crush the garlic.

Place the duck carcass in a large saucepan with the vegetable stock. Add the chicken stock cube and all other ingredients. Bring to the boil, cover the pan and simmer for 1½–2 hours. Taste for flavouring and add another chicken stock cube if necessary.

Strain the soup through a colander to remove all bones, the bay leaves and peppercorns. Allow to cool, then store in a refrigerator. The fat will then separate and rise to the surface. When quite cold, remove all solidified fat from the top of the soup.

Use within 2 days and reheat before serving.

MINESTRONE SOUP

(SERVES 4)

2 sticks celery
2 carrots
1 small cabbage
4 oz (100g) mushrooms
1 medium onion
1 pint (500ml) water
½ pint (250ml) tomato juice
1 teaspoon chilli powder
1 teaspoon mixed dried herbs
salt and freshly ground black pepper

Wash and finely slice the celery. Peel and finely slice the carrots. Trim and shred the cabbage. Wash, trim and chop the mushrooms. Peel and chop the onion and dry-fry in a non-stick frying pan, without any fat. When the onion is soft, place in a large saucepan with the celery, carrots, water, tomato juice and seasonings. Bring to the boil · and simmer for 45 minutes. Add the cabbage and mushrooms and simmer for a further 30 minutes. Adjust seasoning to taste. Serve hot.

MIXED VEGETABLE SOUP

(SERVES 8–10)

8 oz (200g) old but firm potatoes
8 oz (200g) carrots
8 oz (200g) onions
8 oz (200g) leeks
3–4 sticks celery
3½–4½ pints (1.75–2.25 litres) chicken stock
salt and freshly ground black pepper
fresh parsley or chives, chopped, to garnish

Peel the potatoes, carrots and onions. Wash and trim the leeks and celery. Grate the potatoes and carrots and finely slice the onions, leeks and celery. (A food processor or mixer with grating and slicing attachments is ideal for this.)

Place the vegetables in a large pan with 3½ pints (1.75 litres) stock. Season with salt and pepper. Bring to the boil, cover and simmer gently for 20–30 minutes until all the vegetables are tender. If you prefer a smooth soup, purée the vegetables in a food processor or liquidiser or use a vegetable mill.

Add more stock to thin the soup if necessary. Check the seasoning, reheat and pour into a hot soup tureen. Sprinkle the

chopped fresh parsley or chives over the top before serving. Serve hot.

MAIN COURSES: MEAT

BARBECUED KEBABS

(SERVES 4)

1 lb (400g) lean beef or lean boneless pork
Barbecue Sauce (see recipe, page 109), double quantity
1 large onion
1 red pepper
1 green pepper
2 courgettes
mushrooms (optional)
12 cherry tomatoes
4 long, or 8 short, skewers

Cut the beef *or* pork into 1-inch (2.5cm) cubes and marinate in the barbecue sauce for at least one hour, preferably two, before cooking.

Prepare the vegetables by peeling the onion and cutting into medium-sized pieces. Deseed both peppers and cut into squares. Slice the courgettes thickly and trim the mushrooms, if used.

Heat the grill and preheat the skewers. Taking care not to burn your fingers, thread the vegetables and beef *or* pork on to the hot skewers alternately until all the ingredients have been used up or the skewers are full. Brush the kebabs with the remaining barbecue sauce and place under a hot grill to cook, turning them frequently to prevent burning. Place any remaining vegetables on the grill pan to cook, and serve in addition to the kebabs.

When the kebabs are thoroughly cooked, serve them on a bed of boiled rice mixed with beansprouts. Heat any remaining barbecue sauce and serve separately.

BEEFBURGERS

(MAKES APPROXIMATELY 16)

2 lbs (800g) lean beef or finely minced lean beef
2 large onions
1–2 cloves garlic
4 oz (100g) stale bread
2 egg whites
1 teaspoon French mustard
¼ teaspoon allspice
½ teaspoon mixed dried herbs
2 teaspoons salt
black pepper

Mince the beef very finely by passing it through a mincer 2–3 times. If using bought mince, make certain it is very fresh.

Peel the onions and garlic. Chop the onion very finely and crush the garlic, or put them both into a food processor until they are almost puréed.

Soak the bread in a little water for about 5 minutes, then squeeze out.

Whisk the egg whites until frothy.

In a large bowl mix all the ingredients together. It is easier to use your hands for this. If you wish to check the seasoning, dry-fry a small portion of the mixture in a preheated nonstick frying-pan, and taste.

Form the beefburgers either in a mould or by shaping them with wet hands. Layer them with a piece of freezer tissue between each, and store in a plastic box in the freezer. They can then be removed separately.

Dry-fry or grill as required. They will take about 4–5 minutes to cook on each side. Frozen beefburgers need a minute or two longer than fresh ones. Serve with Oven Chips (see recipe, page 134), mushrooms, peas and sweetcorn.

NB This recipe is ideal for barbecues.

FILLET OF BEEF WITH PEPPERCORNS

(SERVES 4)

2 wineglasses white wine
1 tablespoon green peppercorns, drained and rinsed
4 × 6 oz (150g) pieces of beef fillet
6 oz (150g) natural yogurt
freshly ground black pepper

Boil the wine with the peppercorns in a small saucepan until the liquid is reduced by half. Keep it warm while you cook the fillets of beef.

Preheat the grill until it is really hot. Grill the beef fillets for 3 minutes on each side. Lower the grill pan and continue cooking until the fillets are cooked to your taste (rare, medium rare, well done, etc.).

When the steaks are almost ready bring the wine and peppercorn sauce back to boiling point. Remove from the heat and stir into it the natural yogurt, and season to taste. Return the pan to the heat for only a few seconds in order to heat the yogurt through. Do not allow it to boil or it will curdle.

Pour the yogurt, wine and peppercorn sauce over the steaks and serve with unlimited potatoes and other vegetables of your choice.

HAM, BEEF AND CHICKEN OR TURKEY SALAD

(SERVES 4)

6 oz (150g) lean cooked ham
6 oz (150g) lean cooked beef
2 small cooked chicken
breasts or 8 oz (200g) turkey
breast
3 large oranges
2 small heads chicory
1 tablespoon white wine
vinegar or cider vinegar
3 tablespoons lemon juice
salt and black pepper
1 small lettuce
bunch watercress
1–2 tablespoons capers
(optional)

Cut the ham, beef and chicken or turkey into finger-length pieces.

Grate the rind and squeeze the juice from one orange. Cut the peel and pith from the other two oranges and remove the segments or cut into slices. Cut each segment into 2–3 pieces or each slice into quarters.

Wash the chicory. Reserve a few leaves and slice the rest. Mix the vinegar, orange and lemon juice together in a bowl with the grated orange rind. Season with salt and pepper.

Mix the meats, orange pieces and chicory slices together. Line a salad bowl with lettuce leaves. Pile the meat mixture into the centre and arrange the reserved chicory spears standing up around the edge of the bowl. Garnish the top with sprigs of watercress and sprinkle a few capers over it.

LAMB'S LIVER WITH ORANGE

(SERVES 4)

12 oz–1 lb (300–400g) lamb's
liver
¼ pint (125ml) skimmed milk
1 orange, to garnish
salt and freshly ground black
pepper
7 fl oz (175ml) orange juice
¾ teaspoon arrowroot
¼ teaspoon chopped fresh or
powdered thyme

Remove any membrane or veins from the liver. Place in a bowl, pour the skimmed milk over and leave to stand for 1-2 hours if possible, but at least 30 minutes. This will help to keep the liver moist when it is cooked.

Wash and slice the orange. Cut each slice in half. Cover and put to one side.

Dry-fry the liver until it is cooked but slightly pink in the centre, or cook under a preheated grill or on a preheated grillade. When cooked, season with salt and pepper.

Heat the orange juice in a pan. Mix the arrowroot with a little water. Add to the pan and bring to the boil, stirring all the time.

Arrange the liver on a hot dish and pour the sauce over. Sprinkle the thyme over the top and garnish, just before serving, with the orange slices.

Serve hot.

LAMB STEW

(SERVES 4)

3–4 small new turnips
12 small (pickling) onions
8–12 small new carrots
1 lb (400g) small new
potatoes
1¼ lbs (500g) lean boneless
lamb
½ teaspoon caster sugar
1 clove garlic or ½ teaspoon
garlic paste
1½ oz (375g) flour
1 pint (500ml) lamb or
chicken stock
¼ pint (125ml) dry white
wine, cider or extra stock
1 tablespoon tomato purée
salt and black pepper
4 oz (100g) French beans,
fresh or frozen
4 oz (100g) shelled peas, fresh
or frozen
1 tablespoon mixed chopped
parsley and chives

Peel the turnips and cut each into 2 or 4 pieces depending on size. Peel the onions carefully, leaving as much stem and root on as possible to prevent the centres popping out during cooking. Scrape the carrots and potatoes.

Blanch the onions in boiling salted water for 4–5 minutes and the potatoes for 7–8 minutes. Drain, then chill under cold running water. This preserves the fresh taste and the colour of the vegetables. Drain well again.

Trim any fat from the lamb. Cut the meat into 1-inch (2.5cm) dice. Sprinkle with the sugar. Dry-fry in a frying pan or heatproof casserole until golden brown. Remove from the pan.

Peel and crush the garlic. Mix the flour in a small bowl with a little of the stock. Whisk until smooth and add more stock. Pour into the pan with the remainder of the stock and white wine or cider, if used. Bring to the boil, stirring all the time. Add the garlic and the tomato purée. Season to taste with salt and pepper. Return the meat to a heatproof casserole together with the turnips, onions, carrots and potatoes and bring to the boil again. Place in a preheated oven at 170°C, 325°F, or Gas Mark 3 for about 1 hour.

Top and tail fresh French beans and cut into 1-inch (2.5cm) pieces. Blanch fresh beans and fresh peas in boiling salted water for 7–8 minutes. Drain, then chill, as before. Add to the casserole and continue cooking for about another 30 minutes until the meat and vegetables are tender. If using frozen vegetables, allow them to defrost and add to the pan 15–20 minutes before the end of the cooking time.

When the meat and vegetables are tender, taste and adjust the seasoning if necessary. Pour into a hot dish or serve from the casserole. Sprinkle the parsley and chives over before serving.

LIVER AND ONION CASSEROLE

(SERVES 4)

2 large onions
1 lb (400g) liver (lamb's, calves' or ox)
¾ pint (375ml) water
2 beef stock cubes
salt and pepper to taste
1 level tablespoon gravy powder

Peel and slice the onions. Preheat a non-stick frying pan and dry-fry the onions until they turn soft and brown. Remove all membrane from the liver, slice it and add to the onions in the pan. Sauté the liver until it changes colour then add the water and the stock cubes, salt and pepper. Cover the pan and continue cooking on a gentle heat for 20–25 minutes. When the liver is cooked, remove the pan from the heat. Mix the gravy powder with 2 tablespoons of water and add to the pan. Stir thoroughly, then replace the pan on the heat and continue to cook, stirring continuously, for a further 2 or 3 minutes.

Serve immediately with unlimited potatoes and other vegetables of your choice.

MARINADED LAMB

(SERVES 4–5)

4 cloves garlic
3 lbs (1.25kg) knuckle end of leg of lamb
2 teaspoons chopped rosemary
2 teaspoons ground cumin
1 teaspoon chilli powder, or to taste
4 tablespoons red wine vinegar
¼ pint (125ml) red wine or cider

Peel the cloves of garlic. Cut 2

into slivers and crush the other two. With a small sharp knife make deep slits in the lamb and insert the slivers of garlic and some of the rosemary into each one, pressing in well with the point of the knife.

Mix together the crushed cloves of garlic, the remainder of the rosemary, the cumin and chilli powder. Stir in the vinegar, and red wine or cider.

Place the meat in a dish and pour the marinade over. Cover and keep in the refrigerator for 6–8 hours or overnight. Turn the lamb in the marinade several times so that it is well coated.

To cook, drain the meat and place in a roasting tin. Cook in a preheated oven at 180°C, 350°F, or Gas Mark 4 for about 1½ hours until the meat is tender but the juices are slightly pink. If you prefer, you can remove the lamb from the oven after 1 hour, baste well with the marinade and continue cooking over a hot barbecue for a further 40–50 minutes, turning occasionally.

MINI PIZZAS

(MAKES 8)

This recipe will make 8 individual pizzas but if you prefer you can divide the dough and the topping into 2 and make larger pizzas for 4.

If you would rather have wholemeal bread for the base, use 10 oz (250g) wholemeal flour and 6 oz (150g) strong white flour.

For the base
1 lb (400g) packet bread flour mix or 1 lb (400g) strong bread flour
1 sachet easy-to-blend yeast
1 scant teaspoon salt
For the topping
3 large onions
14 oz (350g) tinned chopped tomatoes
1–2 cloves crushed garlic or ½–1 teaspoon garlic paste
½ teaspoon sugar
1–2 teaspoons lemon juice
salt and black pepper
1 tablespoon chopped basil
4 oz (100g) mushrooms
4–6 medium tomatoes
4–6 oz (100–176g) ham

Prepare the bread mix for the base according to the makers' instructions. If making your own, mix the flour, yeast and salt together. Make a well in the centre and pour in 10 fl oz (250ml) tepid water into the centre. Blend in the flour from the sides until it is all incorporated and the dough leaves the sides of the bowl and forms a soft but not sticky ball. Knead for about 5 minutes on a lightly floured board. Return the dough to the bowl, cover with food wrap and leave in a warm place for about 1 hour until doubled in size. Meanwhile make the topping.

Peel and slice the onions and dry-fry until soft and golden brown. Remove 2–3 from the pan and reserve. Add the tinned tomatoes, garlic, sugar and a little lemon juice to the pan. Season well with salt and pepper and cook over a gentle heat until the sauce mixture is quite thick. Stir in the basil.

Slice the mushrooms and tomatoes and coarsely chop the ham.

Divide the bread dough into 8 and knead each piece lightly then roll out into a circle about the size of a saucer. Place the circles on baking sheets. Spread some of the sauce over each piece of dough. Cover with the reserved cooked onions, the ham, mushrooms and tomatoes. Leave for 15–20 minutes until the bread base has risen and bake in a preheated oven at 220°C, 425°F, or Gas Mark 7 for 12–15 minutes until the bread dough and the vegetables are cooked.

NB If you wish, you can open freeze the pizzas at this stage. Place in a plastic bag or box. Seal the container well and store for up to 3 months. Cook from frozen, allowing an extra 5–10 minutes.

SAVOURY MEAT LOAF

....

(SERVES 5–6)

8 oz (200g) lean pork
1 large onion
2 egg whites
1 lb (400g) very lean minced beef
1 tablespoon tomato purée
1 tablespoon chopped parsley
1 tablespoon chopped chives
1 teaspoon fresh chopped thyme or ¼ teaspoon dried thyme
2 oz (50g) fresh brown or white breadcrumbs
1½ teaspoons salt
black pepper

Remove any fat from the pork and peel the onion. Mince together finely.

Lightly whisk the egg whites until they are frothy.

Mix all the ingredients well together until evenly blended. Place in a 2-lb (800g) non-stick loaf tin. Press down well and level the top with a wet tablespoon. Bake in a preheated oven at 190°C, 375°F, or Gas Mark 5 for 1–1¼ hours. If the juices at the side of the tin are pink, continue cooking until they are clear. Cover the top with greaseproof paper if it

starts to brown too much.

Leave until cold. Turn out and slice, and serve with salad or vegetables. If you have difficulty in turning this loaf out of the tin, dip the tin in hot water for a moment or two.

You can, if you wish, serve this meat loaf hot with your favourite home-made tomato sauce or Creole Sauce (see below).

CREOLE SAUCE

1 large onion
1–2 cloves garlic or ½–1 teaspoon garlic paste
1 small green pepper
1 small red pepper
1–2 tablespoons lemon juice
1 teaspoon sugar
10 oz (250g) tomato passata or tinned tomatoes puréed
1 teaspoon French mustard
5 fl oz (125ml) chicken stock, if needed
salt and black pepper
1 tablespoon chopped parsley

Peel the onion and fresh garlic. Finely chop the onion and crush the garlic. Remove the stalk, core, seeds and pith from the peppers and cut the flesh into small dice.

Place the onion, garlic, peppers, 1 tablespoon lemon juice, sugar and the tomato passata or puréed tomatoes in a pan. Stir in the French mustard and season with salt and pepper.

Bring to the boil and simmer gently for 25–30 minutes until the onions and pepper are tender. If the sauce thickens too much during the cooking, add a little chicken stock whilst it is cooking, and adjust the consistency and seasoning when the sauce is cooked. Add the parsley just before serving.

This sauce is also good served with barbecued meats and fish.

SHEPHERD'S PIE

....

(SERVES 4)

1 lb (400g) minced lean beef
½ pint (250ml) water
1 large onion
1 teaspoon mixed herbs
1 teaspoon chilli powder
1 teaspoon gravy powder
1 beef stock cube
1½ lbs (600g) peeled potatoes
salt and freshly ground black pepper

Boil the mince and water in a saucepan for 5 minutes. Drain (reserve the liquid) and keep in a covered container until required. Place the drained liquid in the refrigerator. This will cause any fat to rise to the top and set hard. Remove and discard this.

Peel, chop and dry-fry the onion. When it is soft and brown add the drained mince, herbs and chilli powder and allow to simmer while you re-heat the skimmed liquid in a separate saucepan.

Mix the gravy powder with a little cold water and add the stock cube and skimmed liquid. Bring to the boil, stir-ring continually. Add this gravy to the frying pan, stir well and simmer for a further 10 minutes. Season to taste. The consistency of the mince and gravy should be thick. If it is too thin, allow the liquid to reduce by simmering for longer.

Meanwhile, boil the potatoes until soft. Then drain most, but not all, of the water as the potatoes need to be quite wet for mashing. Mash the potatoes and season well, adding a little skimmed milk from your allowance if neces-sary to make a soft consistency.

Place the mince in an oval ovenproof dish and cover with the mashed potatoes. Place under a preheated grill, to brown the top, or in a hot pre-heated oven for 10 minutes.

Serve hot with unlimited vegetables.

SPICY PORK VOLCANO

(SERVES 4)

16 oz (400g) lean pork
2 large onions
1 green pepper
For the marinade
2 tablespoons tomato ketchup
2 tablespoons brown sauce
1 teaspoon French mustard
5 fl oz (125ml) tomato juice
1 tablespoon soy sauce
salt and freshly ground black pepper
To accompany
8 oz (200g) [dry weight] easy-cook rice
16 oz (400g) tinned beansprouts

Mix all the ingredients for the marinade together. Cut the pork into cubes and leave in the marinade for at least 2 hours.

Peel the onions and deseed the green pepper. Chop both. Dry-fry the onion and green pepper in a non-stick frying pan. When the onion is soft and brown, add the marinated pork, a few pieces at a time, and continue to cook.

When the pork is almost cooked, add any remaining marinade and simmer for a further 5 minutes. Add more tomato juice if the mixture becomes too thick.

Cook the rice in plenty of boiling salted water. When the rice is cooked, strain it through a colander.

Drain the beansprouts and add to the rice in the colander. Pour over them a kettle-full of boiling water, which will heat the beansprouts and rinse the rice.

When the rice is thoroughly drained, mix the beansprouts and the rice together and place on a large serving dish, leaving a well in the middle. Place the pork mixture in the centre and serve immediately.

SPICY SPAGHETTI BOLOGNESE

(SERVES 4)

1 lb (400g) lean minced beef
1 large onion
16 oz (400g) tinned chopped tomatoes
1 tablespoon tomato purée
2 tablespoons tomato ketchup
or 4 fl oz (100ml) tomato juice
1 tablespoon brown sauce
½ teaspoon Tabasco sauce
2 level teaspoons chilli powder
2 cloves garlic, crushed (or ½ teaspoon dried garlic)

Dry-fry the mince in a non-stick frying pan for 10 minutes, stirring frequently, until the meat changes colour. Place the mince in a sieve or fine colander whilst still hot and drain off all the fat.

Peel and chop the onion. Wipe out the frying pan with a piece of kitchen paper and dry-fry the onion until soft and brown. Return the mince to the frying pan with the onion. Add the chopped tomatoes and all other ingredients. Mix well and cover. Cook on a low heat, stirring occasionally, for 45 minutes.

This dish is better if prepared in advance and reheated to serve. Allow 2 oz (50g) un-cooked weight spaghetti per person. Serve with a little Parmesan cheese.

MAIN COURSES: POULTRY AND GAME

BARBECUED CHICKEN KEBABS

(SERVES 2)

2 large chicken joints,
preferably breasts
2 medium-sized onions
1 green pepper
1 red pepper
6 oz (150g) mushrooms
8 bay leaves

BARBECUE SAUCE
2 tablespoons tomato ketchup
2 tablespoons brown sauce
2 tablespoons mushroom
sauce (optional)
2 tablespoons wine vinegar

Cut the chicken flesh into 1-inch (1.2cm) cubes.

Prepare the vegetables by peeling and quartering the onions. Deseed the peppers and cut into bite-sized squares. Wash the mushrooms and leave them whole.

Thread alternate pieces of chicken and vegetables on to 2 skewers to make 2 kebabs, placing a bay leaf on the skewers at intervals to add flavour.

Mix all the sauce ingredients and brush on to the skewered chicken and vegetables, saving any remaining sauce for basting. Leave to marinate for two hours before cooking.

Place kebabs under the grill and cook under a moderate heat, turning them regularly to avoid burning. Baste frequently with the remaining sauce mixture to maintain the moisture. Use no fat.

Serve on a bed of boiled brown rice and grilled fresh tomatoes.

CHICKEN A L'ORANGE

(SERVES 4)

4 chicken breasts
1 wineglass of red wine
3 oranges
1 large Spanish onion
onion salt and white pepper
to taste
1 – 2 tablespoons redcurrant
jelly
2 teaspoons cornflour
¼ pint (125ml) chicken stock

Remove any skin from the chicken breasts and leave to marinate in the red wine for 1 hour. Meanwhile squeeze the juice from the oranges and peel and slice the onion.

Pre-heat a non-stick frying pan and sprinkle with onion salt and white pepper. When the pan is hot, add the chicken pieces (leaving the wine to one side for the moment) and sauté them on a brisk heat until they have changed colour, turning the chicken over to cook both sides. Add the onion or, if there is no room in the pan, dry-fry it in another non-stick frying pan. When the onion has become soft and brown add it to the chicken. Pour in the wine, orange juice and redcurrant jelly. Cover the pan and leave to simmer on a very low heat for 15 minutes or until the chicken is thoroughly cooked.

Meanwhile mix the cornflour with the chicken stock. When the chicken is cooked, remove the chicken pieces from the pan and place on a preheated serving dish to keep warm. Into the pan gradually add the chicken stock and cornflour mixture and mix. Slowly bring to the boil, stirring all the time. Taste and adjust the seasoning to taste.

When ready to serve, pour the orange sauce over the chicken pieces and serve immediately with unlimited potatoes and other vegetables.

CHICKEN AND MUSHROOM SUPREME

(SERVES 4)

freshly ground black pepper
4 chicken breasts
soy sauce
8 oz (200g) button mushrooms
2 teaspoons cornflour
6 tablespoons cold water

Preheat a non-stick frying pan and add a generous amount of freshly ground black pepper. Place the chicken in the hot pan and sprinkle more pepper on to the chicken. Sauté the chicken pieces until they have changed colour on all sides. Cover with a lid, reduce the heat and con-

tinue to cook on a low heat for 20–30 minutes. Add more pepper at approximately 10-minute intervals, at the same time turning the chicken over.

When the chicken is almost cooked add 6 tablespoons soy sauce to the frying pan. Add the button mushrooms, cover and simmer for a further 10 minutes. Add more soy sauce as necessary to prevent the pan becoming too dry.

When the chicken and mushrooms are thoroughly cooked, place them on a preheated serving dish and keep warm.

Add more soy sauce to the frying pan until there is approximately ¼ pint (5 fl oz) fluid. Mix the cornflour and cold water together and carefully stir into the sauce in the pan. Remove from the heat as soon as it begins to thicken and stir vigorously to prevent it becoming lumpy. Return to the heat and cook gently for 2 or 3 minutes.

Serve with hot boiled rice. Place the rice in a preheated serving dish and put the chicken pieces and mushrooms in the centre. Pour the hot sauce over the chicken and mushrooms and serve immediately, with unlimited green vegetables.

CHICKEN AND MUSHROOM PILAFF

(SERVES 4)

8 oz (200g) long-grain brown rice
1½ pints (750ml) chicken stock
6 spring onions
1 clove garlic
2 medium carrots
2 sticks celery
2 tablespoons water
2–3 teaspoons mild curry powder
1 dessertspoon mango chutney
8 oz (200g) cooked chicken, diced
8 oz (200g) open cup mushrooms, wiped and halved
2 tablespoons fresh chopped coriander or parsley
salt and pepper
8 tablespoons low-fat natural yogurt

Cook the rice in chicken stock in a covered saucepan for 25–35 minutes, according to instructions given on the pack. The water should be absorbed but, if not, simmer it uncovered for an extra few minutes.

Prepare the vegetables by chopping the spring onions, crushing the garlic, and slicing the carrots and celery. Place all the vegetables into a saucepan with the water, cover and simmer for 5 minutes. Add the curry powder and cook for 1 minute, then add the chutney, chicken and mushrooms and cook for 3 minutes. Stir in the rice, coriander or parsley, and seasoning. Cook until the rice is reheated.

Serve hot with spoonfuls of yogurt.

CHICKEN AND POTATO CAKES

....

(SERVES 4)

12 oz (300g) chicken meat, cooked
12 oz (300g) potatoes, cooked
2 tablespoons skimmed milk (optional)
1 egg
2 tablespoons fresh parsley, finely chopped
1 teaspoon prepared mustard
salt
freshly ground black pepper

Mince or very finely chop the cooked chicken. Mash the potatoes, adding the milk if they are too dry. Mix together the mashed potato and the chicken.

Add the egg, stir well, then add the parsley, mustard, salt and pepper.

Wet your hands and make chicken and potato cakes.

Dry-fry in a non-stick frying pan until golden brown on each side.

Serve with unlimited vegetables.

CHICKEN AND POTATO PIE

....

(SERVES 4)

1 onion
1 lb (400g) cooked chicken
½ pint (250ml) skimmed milk (in addition to allowance)
1 chicken stock cube
1 bay leaf
6 peppercorns
salt and freshly ground black pepper
1 dessertspoon cornflour
1½ lbs (600g) potatoes, peeled and cooked
2½ oz (62.5g) low-fat natural yogurt

Peel and slice the onion. Chop the chicken coarsely.

Place all but 2 fl oz (50ml) milk in a non-stick saucepan with onion, stock cube, bay leaf and seasonings. Heat gently, then cover the pan. Simmer for five minutes to allow the flavours to infuse. Remove the peppercorns and bay leaf.

Mix the cornflour with the remaining cold milk and gradually add this to the saucepan and stir well. Slowly bring the sauce to the boil, stirring all the time. When boiling gently, add the chopped chicken. The sauce should be a thick creamy consistency. If the sauce is too thin the potato topping will sink. Add more slaked cornflour (i.e. mixed with milk) if necessary to thicken the sauce further. Taste for seasoning and adjust as necessary.

Pour the chicken sauce into a pie dish, allowing space for the potato 'crust' to be added.

Mash the pre-cooked potatoes with yogurt so that the mixture is creamy and light. Add more yogurt or skimmed milk as necessary. Season well. Carefully spoon the potato mixture on to the chicken sauce mixture so that the dish is completely covered to the edges, and smooth over with a fork. Place the dish under a hot grill to brown the top. Serve immediately.

Alternatively, the pie can be made well in advance and then warmed through in a preheated moderate oven (180°C, 350°F, Gas Mark 4) for 20–30 minutes.

CHICKEN CHOP SUEY

(SERVES 4)

4 chicken joints
3 large carrots
5 sticks celery
6 oz (150g) mange tout
(optional)
2 large onions
1 red pepper
2 green peppers
30 oz (750g) beansprouts
4 tablespoons vegetable stock
salt and pepper to taste
soy sauce

Prepare the ingredients as follows. Skin, bone, then coarsely slice the chicken. Peel and coarsely grate the carrots. Finely chop the celery. Trim and wash the mange tout, if using. Peel and finely slice the onions. Deseed all 3 peppers and slice them. Drain the beansprouts.

Add the chicken to the vegetable stock and cook in a large non-stick frying pan or wok on a moderate heat until it changes colour.

Add carrots, onions, celery and mange tout and stir-fry. Add the sliced peppers and beansprouts and continue to cook until thoroughly hot. Season to taste.

Serve on a bed of boiled brown rice, with soy sauce. Allow 1 oz (25g) [dry weight] of rice per person following the diet. Non-slimmers are not restricted.

CHICKEN CURRY

(SERVES 2)

2 chicken joints
1 medium onion
1 eating apple
15 oz (375g) tinned tomatoes
1 bayleaf
2 teaspoons oil-free sweet pickle or Branston pickle
1 teaspoon tomato purée
1 tablespoon curry powder

Remove all fat and skin from the chicken joints. Chop the onion finely. Core the apple and chop into small pieces.

Place all the ingredients in a saucepan and bring to the boil. Cover and cook slowly for about 1 hour, stirring occasionally and turning the chicken joints every 15 minutes or so. If the mixture is too thin, remove the lid and cook on a slightly higher heat until the sauce reduces and thickens.

Serve on a bed of boiled brown rice.

CHICKEN FRICASSEE

(SERVES 4)

1 pint (500ml) skimmed milk
(in addition to allowance)
6 peppercorns
2 bay leaves
2 slices onion
1 chicken stock cube
2 dessertspoons cornflour
3 tablespoons water
salt and pepper
4 cooked chicken breasts

Bring the milk, peppercorns, bay leaves, onion and stock cube to the boil. Cover the pan with a lid, remove from heat and let it stand for 15–20 minutes to infuse.

Strain the milk into another pan, bring almost to boiling point, then remove from the heat. Mix the cornflour and water and stir into the milk. Return the pan to the heat and slowly bring to boiling point, stirring all the time. Season to taste.

Chop the chicken coarsely, add to the sauce and continue cooking on a low heat for 5 minutes.

Serve with unlimited vegetables of your choice.

CHICKEN ITALIENNE

....

(SERVES 4)

2 cloves garlic
freshly ground black pepper
1 teaspoon dried oregano
1½ lbs (600g) chicken flesh,
without skin
1 red pepper
1 green pepper
1 large onion
2 tablespoons tomato purée
16 oz (400g) tinned chopped
tomatoes
chicken stock cube
10 oz (250g) spaghetti

Peel and crush the garlic. Preheat a non-stick frying pan and sprinkle with the black pepper, garlic and oregano. Finely slice the chicken and add to the pan. Sprinkle the chicken with more black pepper and cook until it changes colour.

Deseed and finely chop both peppers. Peel and chop the onion. Add the peppers and onion to the pan and continue cooking, stirring frequently to prevent the vegetables from burning. When the onion begins to turn brown, add the tomato purée and the chopped tomatoes. Mix well and add more freshly ground black pepper. Cover the pan with a lid and continue cooking for a further 10 minutes.

Meanwhile, dissolve the chicken stock cube in a pan of boiling water, add the spaghetti and bring back to the boil.

As soon as the spaghetti is cooked, drain it and serve immediately with the chicken sauce.

CHICKEN PILAFF

....

(SERVES 4)

1 large onion
1 green pepper
1 pint (500ml) water
8 oz (200g) long-grain rice
2 chicken stock cubes
12 oz (300g) chicken
5 fl oz (125ml) white wine
salt and pepper
4 oz (100g) frozen peas
10–12 oz (250–300g) canned
sweetcorn

Peel the onion and chop finely. Cook in a non-stick frying pan until soft and brown. Deseed the green pepper, chop it finely and add it to the pan and continue dry-frying.

Meanwhile, bring the water to boil in a large saucepan. Stir in the rice and the stock cubes. Continue cooking on a moderate heat until all the water has been absorbed and the rice is cooked. Stir frequently and add a little water as necessary to prevent sticking.

Skin, bone and chop the chicken into ½-inch (1.25cm) strips. Once the onion and pepper are cooked add the chicken and continue cooking. When the chicken has changed colour, add the wine and cook for a further 5 minutes. Sprinkle liberally with freshly ground black pepper, and salt if liked.

Lightly cook the peas and sweetcorn (these can be cooked together in one pan). Drain the peas and sweetcorn and add to the frying pan immediately. Stir the chicken-flavoured boiled rice into the chicken and vegetables. Serve straightaway in a large preheated serving dish.

NB Do not rinse the rice after cooking as to do so would rinse away the chicken flavour.

CHICKEN WITH ORANGE AND APRICOTS

....

(SERVES 4)

1 onion
2 large oranges
5 fl oz (125ml) orange juice
5 fl oz (125ml) dry white wine or cider
1 teaspoon arrowroot
4 chicken breasts or quarters
salt and pepper
8 oz (225g) fresh apricots or tinned apricots in natural juice
1 tablespoon chopped chervil or parsley

Peel the onion and chop finely. Peel the rind from 1 orange very thinly and cut into fine (julienne) strips. Blanch in a little boiling water for 4–5 minutes until tender. Drain but reserve the water. Reserve the strips of peel for garnishing. Cut away the pith from this orange and then cut out the orange segments. Grate the rind from the other orange and squeeze the juice.

Place the chopped onion in a pan with all the orange juice and the white wine or cider. Simmer gently until tender. Make the liquid up to ½ pint (300ml) with the reserved liquid. Mix the arrowroot with a little water and add to the pan. Bring to the boil, stirring all the time.

Skin the chicken and place in an ovenproof casserole. Pour the sauce over and season to taste with salt and pepper. Cover and cook in a preheated oven at 180°C, 350°F, or Gas Mark 4 for about 30–35 minutes until the chicken is almost tender.

Halve the fresh apricots and remove the stones, or drain the tinned apricots. Add to the casserole and continue cooking for a further 10–20 minutes until the chicken and fruit are tender. Add the reserved orange segments about 5 minutes before the end of the cooking time so that they just heat through.

Check the seasoning. Pour into a hot dish or serve from the casserole. Sprinkle the strips of peel and the chervil or parsley over the top just before serving.

COQ AU VIN

....

(SERVES 4)

3½–4 lbs (1.4–1.6kg) roasting chicken
4 oz (100g) back bacon, with all fat removed
4 oz (100g) button onions
7 fl oz (175ml) red wine (preferably Burgundy)
2 cloves garlic, crushed with ½ teaspoon salt
bouquet garni
¼–½ pint (125–250ml) chicken stock
salt and pepper
1 teaspoon cornflour
3 tablespoons water
chopped parsley, to garnish
French loaf

Joint and skin the chicken and place in a non-stick frying pan. Over a fairly brisk heat, brown the chicken all over and then remove to one side while other ingredients are prepared. Cut the bacon into strips, approximately 1½ inches (3.75cm) long, and blanch these and the onions by putting them in a pan of cold water, bringing to the boil and draining well.

Put the onions and bacon into the frying pan over a brisk heat until they are brown. Replace the chicken joints and pour over the wine. Bring to the

Right: Coq au Vin

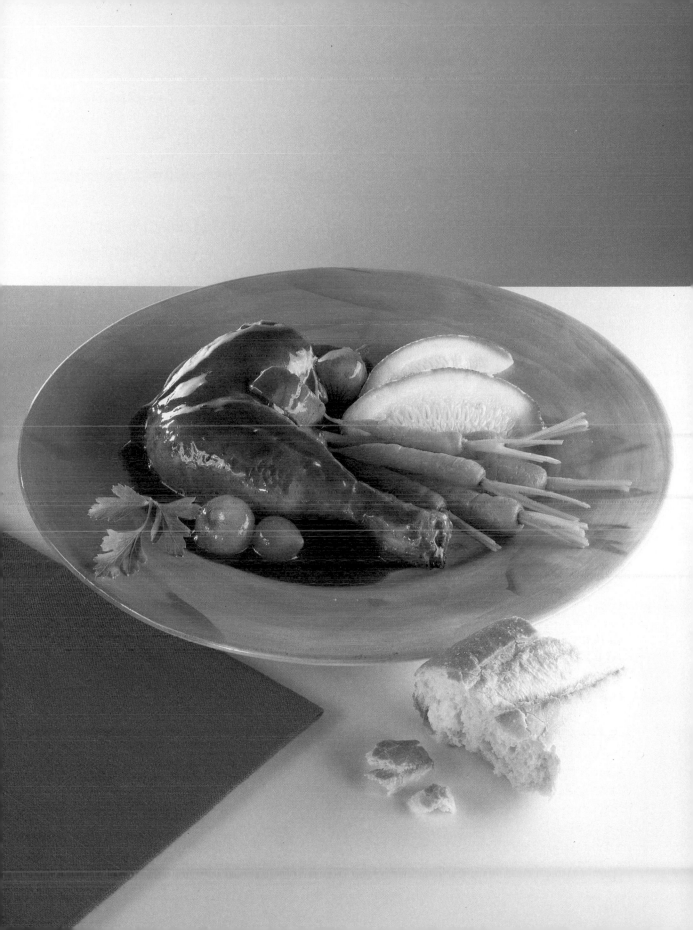

boil and 'flame' by setting the pan alight with a match. This removes the alcohol from the wine.

Add the crushed garlic, bouquet garni, stock and seasoning. Cover the pan and cook slowly for about 1 hour, or place in a casserole and put in a preheated oven at 170°C, 325°F, or Gas Mark 3.

Test to see that the chicken is tender and that it is thoroughly cooked. Discard the bouquet garni, remove the chicken to one side and keep warm. Mix the cornflour and water to a smooth paste. Slowly pour this into the sauce, stirring continuously to keep it smooth. Return to the heat and boil, stirring all the time. Place the chicken pieces back into the casserole and pour the sauce over. Garnish with parsley and serve immediately with slices of French bread.

CURRIED CHICKEN AND YOGURT SALAD

....

(See page 94)

CHINESE CHICKEN SALAD

....

(SERVES 4)

12 oz (300g) cooked chicken breast
4 oz (100g) canned water chestnuts
4 oz (100g) fresh beansprouts
4 spring onions
4 oz (100g) mange tout
5 oz (125g) low-fat natural yogurt
2 teaspoons freshly squeezed lemon juice
2 cloves garlic, crushed
½ teaspoon finely minced fresh ginger or ¼ teaspoon dry ginger
salt and pepper to taste

Prepare the ingredients by finely chopping the chicken and water chestnuts. Wash the beansprouts and peel and chop the spring onions. Blanch the mange tout by putting them in a pan of cold water, bringing them to the boil and draining well.

Mix together in a large bowl the chicken, beansprouts, water chestnuts, mange tout and spring onions. In a smaller bowl mix together the yogurt, lemon juice, garlic and ginger and season to taste. Stir the dressing into the chicken mixture and keep chilled until ready to serve.

Line a large serving bowl with green salad and place the Chinese chicken salad in the centre. Garnish with watercress, if liked.

GLAZED CHICKEN

....

(SERVES 4)

4 chicken breasts, part-boned, or 8 chicken thighs
1 teaspoon French mustard
3 tablespoons tomato ketchup
1 tablespoon honey
1 tablespoon soy sauce
1 tablespoon lemon juice
¾ teaspoon ground ginger
2–3 drops Tabasco sauce or good pinch cayenne pepper
½ pint (250ml) chicken stock
1 teaspoon arrowroot
watercress
lemon wedges

Remove the skin from the chicken and make cuts in the flesh about ½ inch (1.25cm) apart. Place in a shallow dish.

Mix together the mustard, tomato ketchup, honey, soy sauce, lemon juice, ground ginger and Tabasco sauce or cayenne pepper. Spoon the mixture over the chicken pieces, cover and refrigerate for 3–4 hours. Spoon the marinade over the chicken occasionally.

Remove the chicken from the dish and place in a non-stick roasting tin. Reserve the rest of the marinade. Cook the chicken in a preheated oven at 190°C, 375°F, or Gas Mark 5 for 25–30 minutes until tender. Arrange on a hot serving dish.

Stir the stock into the remainder of the marinade and mix well. Pour into a saucepan and bring to the boil. Mix the arrowroot with a little water and add to the pan. Bring to the boil again, stirring all the time.

Garnish the chicken with watercress and lemon wedges. Serve the sauce separately.

HOT CHICKEN SURPRISE

....
(SERVES 4)

freshly ground black pepper
4 chicken breasts with all skin removed
8 oz (200g) brown rice
1 lb (400g) canned beansprouts
soy sauce

Preheat a non-stick frying pan and sprinkle generously with freshly ground black pepper. When the pan is hot, add the chicken pieces and sauté until they change colour and begin to brown. Sprinkle liberally with more black pepper and turn the chicken pieces over to cook the other side. Reduce the heat, cover the pan with a lid and continue cooking for 20 minutes on a low heat, turning the chicken pieces over every 5 minutes or so. The steam trapped by covering the pan prevents the chicken from burning.

Meanwhile, cook the rice in boiling water and drain.

When ready to serve, drain the canned beansprouts and mix them together with the rice in a colander. Pour over a kettle-full of boiling water to reheat the rice and beansprouts. Drain well and place on a preheated serving dish. Top with the chicken pieces and serve with soy sauce to taste.

INDIAN CHICKEN

....
(SERVES 4)

4 chicken breasts
1 chicken stock cube dissolved in ¼ pint (125ml) water
1 dessertspoon curry powder
1 clove garlic, crushed with ½ teaspoon salt
For the rice
4 oz (100g) long grain rice
1 small onion
4 oz (100g) lean ham
1 tablespoon fresh mixed herbs
salt and freshly ground black pepper
1 egg, beaten

For the sauce
½ pint (250ml) skimmed milk (in addition to allowance), brought to the boil with a slice of onion, 1 bay leaf and 6 peppercorns, and left to stand for at least 15 minutes
salt and pepper
1 dessertspoon cornflour

Cook the rice in boiling water and drain.

Peel and chop the onion and dry-fry in a non-stick pan until soft.

Chop the ham and place in a basin with the cooked rice and mixed herbs. Mix in the onion and seasonings and bind with the beaten egg. Place the rice mixture in an ovenproof dish, cover and set aside until needed.

Heat a non-stick frying pan and when hot add the chicken breasts. Brown them on both sides, turning occasionally to prevent burning. When half-cooked, add half the chicken stock, all the curry powder and crushed garlic. Cover the pan and allow to simmer for 20 minutes. Turn the chicken occasionally and add extra stock if the pan becomes dry.

Meanwhile, begin preparing the sauce. Allow the milk and seasonings to infuse. Mix the cornflour with a little milk and add it to the strained warm (not hot) milk. Do not reheat yet.

When the chicken breasts are almost cooked, remove them from the pan, saving any liquid for the sauce. Place the chicken on top of the prepared rice mixture, cover with tin foil and place in a preheated oven at 180°C, 350°F, or Gas Mark 4 for 20 minutes.

Pour any remaining stock into the frying pan and boil up well. Pour into the sauce mixture and stir well. Season to taste. Bring the sauce slowly to the boil just prior to serving, stirring continuously. It should be the consistency of gravy, so adjust by adding more skimmed milk or slaked corn-flour as necessary. The sauce should be a yellow colour.

When ready to serve, remove the covering from the rice and chicken dish and pour the sauce over the chicken pieces and rice. Serve with green vegetables of your choice, such as peas, beans or broccoli spears.

ROSY DUCK SALAD

(SERVES 4–6)

4½ lbs (1.8kg) cold roasted duck
2 oranges
5 tablespoons low-fat fromage frais
2 tablespoons tomato ketchup
1–2 teaspoons curry powder
1 teaspoon French mustard
salt and white pepper
6–8 very small tomatoes
1 pink grapefruit
½ small red pepper
½ small yellow pepper
a small selection of red salads, e.g. ½ lollo rosso, ½ oak-leaved lettuce, plus a little raddichio
a few nasturtium flowers (optional)

Remove the skin from the duck and cut the meat into small strips.

Grate the rind from one orange. Remove the rind and pith from both oranges and cut out the segments. Mix the duck with the orange segments and grated rind.

Mix the fromage frais with the tomato ketchup, curry powder and mustard. Season and carefully fold about half into the duck and the orange segments.

Wash the tomatoes. Cut the peel and pith from the grape-fruit and cut out the segments. Remove the core, pith and seeds from the peppers and cut into thin strips.

Arrange some of the red-leaved salad on a serving dish. Pile the duck and orange mixture in the centre and garnish with the grapefruit segments, 3–4 tomatoes, a few strips of pepper and the nasturtium flowers, if used. Serve the rest of the salad in a separate bowl. Also serve the rest of the sauce separately. Refrigerate until required.

SAVOURY OVEN-BAKED CHICKEN LEGS

(SERVES 4)

8 chicken legs
2 tablespoons flour
1 teaspoon salt
¼ teaspoon black pepper
4–6 tablespoons browned breadcrumbs (see note at end of recipe)
1 tablespoon chopped parsley
½ teaspoon chopped fresh or dried rosemary
grated rind of 1 lemon
2 egg whites
2 tablespoons reduced-oil salad dressing (any brand)

Remove the skin from the chicken legs.

Combine the flour, salt and

black pepper in a plastic bag.

Combine the browned breadcrumbs with the parsley, rosemary and grated lemon rind in another bag.

Whisk the egg whites until lightly frothy and mix with the reduced-oil salad dressing.

To coat the chicken legs, place one or two of them in the bag with the flour and shake until coated. Then coat them with the egg white mixture. You may find it easier to use a pastry brush to make certain they are completely coated. Shake off any surplus liquid and put them in the bag with the breadcrumbs and shake until coated. Repeat until all the chicken legs are coated.

Place in a non-stick roasting tin and bake in a preheated oven at 190°C, 375°F, or Gas Mark 5 for 25–30 minutes until cooked through and golden brown. Eat hot, or allow to cool and eat cold with a salad.

NB Chicken joints and thighs can be coated in the same way, but allow an extra 5–10 minutes cooking time for chicken thighs and an extra 15 minutes for chicken pieces.

BROWNED BREADCRUMBS
Although you can use commercially-made breadcrumbs, you may find that home-made ones

are finer and nicer. Start by making ordinary brown or white breadcrumbs in the usual way, then place them in a thin layer in a large roasting tin. Bake them in a moderate oven until they are lightly browned, shaking the tin occasionally until they are evenly coloured. Place in a food processor or liquidiser to break down the breadcrumbs to a fine texture. If you wish, you can then sieve them to take out the coarser pieces. Return these to the food processor until they are fine. These breadcrumbs will keep for several months in an airtight container or in the deep-freeze.

STIR-FRIED CHICKEN AND VEGETABLES

....

(SERVES 1)

4 oz (100g) chicken
15 oz (375g) tinned beansprouts
1 Spanish onion
3 oz (75g) mushrooms
3 sticks celery
1 oz (25g) [dry weight] brown rice

Remove the skin from the chicken and slice coarsely. Prepare the vegetables. Drain the beansprouts, peel the onion and wash, trim and finely slice

the mushrooms. Finely slice the celery and onion.

Partly cook the chicken in a non-stick frying pan or wok until it changes colour. Add the prepared vegetables, a little at a time, until all ingredients are cooked. Stir well while cooking. For best results the vegetables should be only lightly cooked.

Serve with boiled brown rice.

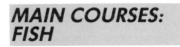

MAIN COURSES: FISH

BARBECUED FISH KEBABS

....

(SERVES 4)

1 lb 4 oz (500g) cod or halibut steak
Barbecue Sauce (see recipe, page 109), double quantity
1 large onion
1 red pepper
1 green pepper
2 courgettes
mushrooms (optional)
12 cherry tomatoes (optional)
4 long or 8 short skewers

Cut the fish steaks into 1-inch (2.5cm) cubes and marinate in the barbecue sauce for at least one hour, preferably two, before cooking.

Prepare the vegetables by peeling the onion and cutting it into medium-sized pieces. Deseed both peppers and cut them into squares. Slice the courgettes thickly and trim the mushrooms if used.

Heat the grill and preheat the skewers if they are metal ones. Taking care not to burn your fingers, thread the vegetables and fish on to the hot skewers alternately until all the ingredients have been used up or the skewers are full. Brush the kebabs with the remaining barbecue sauce and place under a hot grill to cook, turning them frequently to prevent burning. Place any remaining vegetables on the grill pan to cook, and serve in addition to the kebabs.

When the kebabs are thoroughly cooked, serve them on a bed of boiled rice cooked in water with a fish stock cube. Heat any remaining barbecue sauce and serve separately.

To vary this menu, try chicken, pork or beef in place of fish.

COLD PRAWN AND RICE SALAD

....

(SERVES 4)

1 lb (400g) long grain rice
1 lb (400g) prepared prawns
or shrimps
6 tablespoons Citrus Dressing
(see recipe, page 146)
For the sauce
2 small onions, finely chopped
16 oz (400g) tinned, chopped
tomatoes
1 level tablespoon curry
powder
2 tablespoons mango chutney
1 teaspoon sugar
salt to taste
1 teaspoon cornflour
8 tablespoons reduced-oil
salad dressing (any brand)
5 oz (125g) low-fat natural
yogurt
few drops Tabasco sauce
1 teaspoon lemon juice
fresh parsley, to decorate

Boil the rice in plenty of salted water until just tender. Drain and rinse well in cold water and keep in the refrigerator until required.

Gently sauté the chopped onion in a non-stick frying pan. Cook until soft, but not coloured. Tip in the chopped tomatoes and add the curry powder, chutney, sugar and salt. Slake the cornflour in two tablespoons cold water and add to the mixture. Stir well and slowly bring to the boil, stirring continuously, then simmer gently for 30 minutes. Rub the mixture through a sieve into a bowl and leave to cool.

Mix the purée with reduced-oil salad dressing, yogurt, Tabasco and lemon juice. Adjust seasoning to taste and stir in the prawns or shrimps. Place in a refrigerator until required.

To serve, using a fork, blend the Citrus Dressing into the rice and place it in a large oval dish, piling it up towards the rim. Spoon the prawn or shrimp filling into the centre and decorate with parsley. Serve with a green salad.

COD PARCELS

....

(SERVES 4)

1½ lbs (600g) cod or haddock
salt and pepper
1 clove fresh garlic
2 tablespoons lemon juice
3 fl oz (75ml) water
8 spring onions

Divide the fish into 4 equal-sized steaks. Place each steak on a square of aluminium tin foil that is large enough to fold over to make a parcel. Sprinkle the fish with salt and pepper.

Crush the garlic and mix

with the lemon juice and water. Chop the spring onions and add to the liquid. Place equal amounts on to each portion of fish and fold the foil to make a secure parcel.

Place on a baking try and bake in a preheated oven at 190°C, 375°F, or Gas Mark 5.

Serve with unlimited vegetables of your choice.

FISH CAKES

(SERVES 4)

12 oz (300g) potatoes
1 lb (400g) cod
1 egg white
2 tablespoons fresh parsley, finely chopped
1 teaspoon prepared mustard
salt and freshly ground black pepper

Peel the potatoes and boil for 15–20 minutes until cooked. Meanwhile, bake, steam or microwave the cod until cooked. Remove any skin or bones from the fish and flake it. Drain the potatoes and mash until smooth. Mix the fish and potatoes together. Add the egg white and stir well. Add the parsley, mustard, salt and pepper and mix again. Wet your hands and make fish cakes by shaping the mixture into small balls and gently flattening

them. Dry-fry in a non-stick frying pan until golden brown on each side. Serve with un-limited vegetables.

FISH CURRY

(SERVES 4)

2 eating apples
1 large onion
15 oz (375g) tinned tomatoes
1 bay leaf
2 tablespoons oil-free sweet pickle or Branston pickle
2 tablespoons tomato purée
2 tablespoons curry powder
6 tablespoons tomato juice
2 cloves garlic, crushed
4 × 8oz (4 × 200g) pieces frozen haddock

Core the apples and chop them into small pieces. Finely chop the onion. Place all the ingredients except the fish in a saucepan and bring to the boil. Cover and cook slowly for about 20 minutes, stirring occasionally.

Cut the fish into chunks and add to the mixture. Cook for a further 10 minutes.

If the mixture is too thin, re-move the lid and cook on a slightly higher heat until the sauce reduces and thickens.

Serve on a bed of boiled brown rice.

FISH PIE

(SERVES 4)

1½ lbs (600g) cod
salt and pepper
1½ lbs (600g) potatoes

Bake, steam or microwave the fish but do not overcook. Season well.

Boil the potatoes until well done and mash with a little cold water to make a soft consistency. Season well.

Place fish in an ovenproof dish. Flake the flesh, remove the skin, and distribute the fish evenly across the base of the dish. Cover the fish completely with the mashed potatoes and smooth over with a fork.

If the ingredients are still hot just place under a hot grill for a few minutes to brown the top. Alternatively, the pie can be made well in advance and then warmed through in a preheated moderate oven at 180°C, 350°F, or Gas Mark 4 for 20 minutes, or microwaved on high for 5 minutes.

NICOISE SALAD

....

(SERVES 4)

12 oz (300g) new potatoes
8 oz (200g) French beans
4 medium-sized tomatoes
8 oz (200g) tinned tuna fish in brine
4 anchovy fillets (optional)
2–3 tablespoons oil-free vinaigrette
1 small lettuce
a few capers (optional)
1–2 hard-boiled eggs

Scrape the new potatoes and cook in boiling salted water until tender. Drain and chill under cold running water. Drain well again and slice or dice the potatoes.

Top and tail the French beans and cut each one into 2–3 pieces. Cook in boiling salted water for 8–10 minutes until only just tender. Chill and drain as above.

Peel the tomatoes and cut into quarters. Drain the tuna fish and break into chunks. Wash the anchovy fillets in cold water and cut in half lengthways.

Mix together the potatoes, French beans, tomatoes, tuna fish and the oil-free vinaigrette.

Line a dish or bowl with lettuce leaves. Pile the mixture in the centre. Garnish the top with the strips of anchovy, if used. Sprinkle the capers over the top and arrange thin wedges of egg around the outside of the fish mixture. Cover and refrigerate until required.

ORIENTAL PRAWN SALAD

....

(SERVES 6)

6 oz (150g) easy-to-cook rice
1 fish stock cube (optional)
2 oz (50g) mixed red and green peppers, chopped
2 oz (50g) cooked peas
2 oz (50g) cooked sweetcorn
4 tablespoons oil-free vinaigrette
salt and pepper
1 small cucumber
4 tomatoes
½ bunch spring onions
5 oz (125g) low-fat natural yogurt
2 tablespoons tomato ketchup
1–2 teaspoons curry powder
1 small lettuce
1–1½ lbs (400–600g) prawns
4–6 whole prawns

Rinse the rice and cook with the stock cube according to the instructions on the packet. Leave until cold then mix with the peppers, peas, sweetcorn and the oil-free vinaigrette. Season to taste if necessary and arrange in a ring around the sides of a flat dish.

Meanwhile, cut off one-quarter of the cucumber and reserve. Peel the remaining three-quarters and slice in half lengthways. Remove the seeds with a ball-cutter or teaspoon and cut the flesh into small dice. Sprinkle a little salt over and leave for about 30 minutes then rinse and drain well.

Peel and deseed one tomato. Cut into dice. Thinly slice the remainder of the cucumber and tomatoes. Cut each slice in half. Trim and thinly slice the spring onions.

Mix together the yogurt and tomato ketchup and curry powder to taste. Season well.

Wash the lettuce and drain well. Garnish each end of the dish with lettuce and finely shred the rest.

Make certain the prawns are completely defrosted. Rinse and drain them well. Mix together with the shredded lettuce, diced cucumber, diced tomato and the spring onions. Stir in the yogurt mixture and check the seasoning. Remove the shells from the tails of the whole prawns, leaving the heads intact.

Pile the prawn mixture into the centre of the rice. Arrange half slices of tomato and cucumber alternately around the dish, and place the whole prawns in the centre. Cover and refrigerate until required.

POACHED TROUT WITH CUCUMBER SAUCE

....

(SERVES 4)

1 carrot
1 small onion
3–4 cloves
1 bay leaf
sprig fresh thyme
a few parsley stalks
2 tablespoons white wine
vinegar or cider vinegar
½ pint (250ml) water
1 teaspoon salt
white pepper
4 × 8 oz (200g) trout
½ cucumber, to garnish

Peel the carrot and onion. Slice the carrot thinly. Cut the onion in two and stick 2 cloves into each piece.

Place the carrot and onion in a pan with the bay leaf, fresh thyme, parsley stalks, white wine vinegar or cider vinegar and ½ pint (250ml) water. Add the salt and a little white pepper and bring to the boil. Simmer gently for 20–30 minutes. This is called a court bouillon.

Meanwhile, scrape the scales from the trout with a small sharp knife and cut off the fins with scissors. Place in a heat-proof dish.

Pour the court bouillon over the fish, cover with lid and cook for 5 minutes over a gentle heat. Remove the fish carefully from the dish and take off the skins. Return the fish to the dish, replace the lid and continue cooking for another 7–8 minutes after the liquid comes to the boil. Leave in the court bouillon until cold.

Remove the trout from the dish and allow them to drain, then arrange on a serving dish. Finely slice the cucumber and arrange around the sides of the dish. Serve with a green salad and cucumber sauce.

CUCUMBER SAUCE

½ small cucumber
salt
1 shallot or small onion (a pickling onion is ideal)
3–4 tablespoons lemon juice
2–3 tablespoons low-fat fromage frais or low-fat natural yogurt
3–4 drops Tabasco sauce

Peel the cucumber and cut in half lengthways. Remove the seeds with a ball-cutter or teaspoon and cut the flesh into dice. Sprinkle with a little salt and leave for 30–40 minutes then rinse well and spread on kitchen paper to dry.

Peel and coarsely chop the shallot or onion.

Purée the cucumber and shallot or onion in a food processor or liquidiser with lemon juice and fromage frais or yogurt.

Season to taste with Tabasco sauce, and a little salt if necessary, and add more lemon juice and fromage frais or yogurt to suit your taste.

Pour into a sauceboat. Cover and chill before serving.

PRAWN PILAFF

....

(SERVES 4)

1 lb (800g) peeled prawns, fresh or frozen
1 pint (500ml) water
8 oz (200g) long-grain rice
2 fish stock cubes
1 large onion
1 green pepper
5 fl oz (250ml) white wine
salt and pepper
4 oz (100g) frozen peas
10–12 oz (250–300g) canned sweetcorn

If you are using frozen prawns allow time for them to defrost completely. Rinse and drain the prawns, whether fresh or defrosted.

Bring the water to boil in a large saucepan and stir in the rice and the stock cubes. Continue cooking on a moderate heat until all the water has been absorbed and the rice is cooked. Stir frequently and add a little water as necessary to prevent sticking.

Meanwhile, peel the onion

and deseed the pepper and chop both finely. Dry-fry the onion in a non-stick frying pan until soft and brown. Add the green pepper and continue dry-frying until cooked. Add the wine and prawns and continue cooking for 5 minutes. Sprinkle liberally with salt and black pepper.

Lightly cook the peas and sweetcorn (these can be cooked together in one pan). Drain the peas and sweetcorn and add to the frying pan immediately. Stir the fish-flavoured boiled rice into the prawns and vegetables.

Serve immediately in a large preheated serving dish.

NB Do not rinse the rice after cooking as to do so would rinse away the fish stock flavour.

PRAWN STIR-FRY

(SERVES 4)

6 sticks celery
3 carrots
1 medium onion
15 oz (375g) canned or 8 oz (200g) fresh beansprouts
1 lb (400g) shelled prawns
soy sauce
freshly ground black pepper

Wash and chop the celery. Peel the carrots and onion, and coarsely grate both. If using tinned beansprouts, drain well.

Using a wok or non-stick frying pan, carefully cook all the ingredients together, tossing them regularly to avoid burning. The juices from the vegetables will prevent them sticking to the pan. Ensure that the prawns are thoroughly cooked.

Serve with boiled brown rice and extra soy sauce.

TROUT WITH APPLES

(SERVES 4)

4 large trout
1 large or 2 small eating apples
1 small onion
2 oz (50g) brown breadcrumbs
2 tablespoons lemon juice
salt and freshly ground black pepper
4 fl oz (100ml) natural apple juice
2 tablespoons orange juice

Ask your fishmonger to gut the trout for you. Finish preparing the trout at home as follows. Scrape the scales from the trout with a sharp knife and place on a board with the gutted side downwards. Press down along the backbone to ease it away from the flesh. Turn the fish over and remove the backbone and any remaining bones. Use scissors to cut the backbone away from the trout near the tail and head. Remove any fins with the scissors. Rinse under the tap to wash away unwanted loose scales or bones.

Core the apple(s) and peel and grate the apple(s) and onion. Mix together the onion, apple, breadcrumbs and lemon juice and season with salt and pepper.

Sprinkle the inside of each fish with black pepper then fill evenly with the apple stuffing. Close the flesh of the fish around the stuffing.

Place the fish in an ovenproof dish and pour over the apple juice and orange juice. Cover with aluminium foil and bake in a preheated oven at 180°C, 350°F, or Gas Mark 4 for about 40–45 minutes. Sprinkle the chopped parsley on the top just before serving.

Serve hot with potatoes creamed with natural yogurt and any vegetables of your choice.

Right: Prawn Stir-Fry

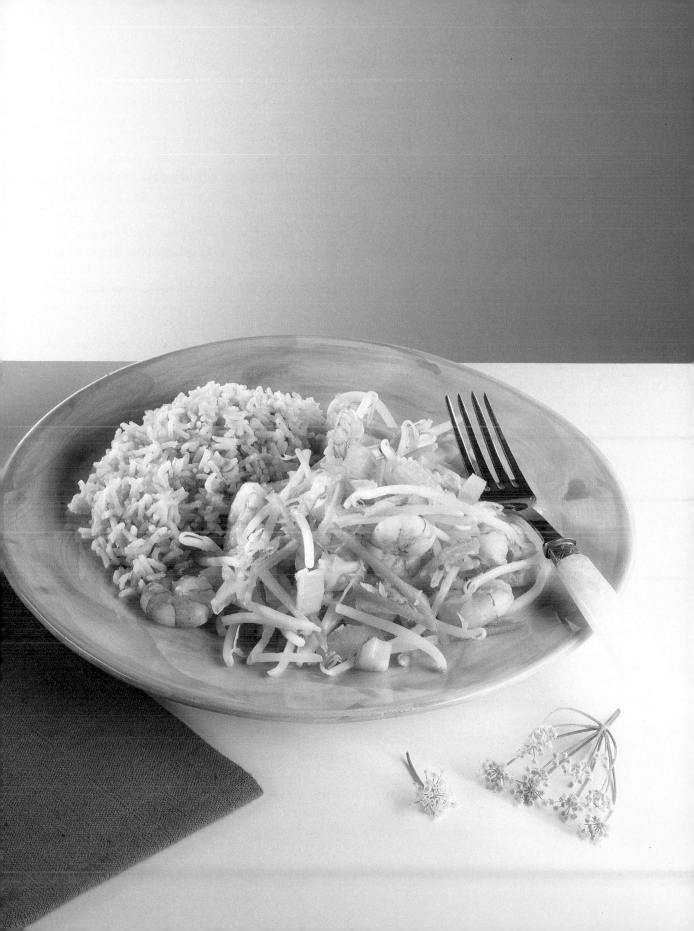

MAIN COURSES: VEGETARIAN

BEAN AND VEGETABLE BAKE

(SERVES 4)

8 oz (200g) carrots
1 lb (400g) white cabbage
1 small cauliflower
1 onion
8 oz (200g) mushrooms
1½ lbs (600g) potatoes
1 lb (400g) tinned baked beans
15 oz (375g) tinned chopped tomatoes
1 tablespoon mixed herbs
salt and freshly ground black pepper
1 tablespoon Parmesan cheese

Prepare the vegetables. Peel and dice the carrots, shred the cabbage and trim and chop the cauliflower. Peel and slice the onion, wash, trim and slice the mushrooms and either peel or scrub the potatoes and slice them. In one pan boil the carrots and cauliflower for 5 minutes. In another pan boil the potatoes for 15 minutes. In a third pan boil the onion and cabbage for 5 minutes.

Place the carrots, half the mushrooms and all the beans into a large casserole or lasagne dish. Place the onion and shredded cabbage on top, followed by the chopped tomatoes, herbs, salt and plenty of black pepper. Cover with the cauliflower and sliced potato. Place the remaining mushrooms on top of the sliced potatoes. Sprinkle on the Parmesan cheese and more black pepper. Place in a pre-heated oven at 150°C, 300°F, or Gas Mark 2 for 30 minutes or until the vegetables are cooked.

Serve immediately.

BLACKEYE BEAN CASSEROLE

(SERVES 4)

4 oz (100g) blackeye beans
1 large onion
6 oz (150g) mushrooms (optional)
3 oz (75g) potato
8 oz (200g) celery
6 oz (150g) carrots
2 oz (50g) water chestnuts (optional)
1 teaspoon chilli powder
½ teaspoon ground ginger (optional)
1 clove garlic, crushed
½ pint (250ml) cold vegetable stock
1 dessertspoon cornflour
1 tablespoon soy sauce
freshly ground black pepper

Cook the blackeye beans in plenty of water for 30–35 minutes by bringing to the boil and then simmering in a covered pan.

Prepare the vegetables by peeling and slicing the onion. Trim and slice the mushrooms, if used. Peel the potato and cut into thin strips. Cut the celery and carrots into thin strips. Slice the water chestnuts thinly, if used.

Gently heat the vegetables, chilli, ginger and garlic in a little stock for 10 minutes. Mix the cornflour and soy sauce in a separate container with a little stock and then stir in remainder of the stock. Add this mixture to the vegetables and then add the drained beans. Simmer for 8–10 minutes and season to taste.

Serve on a bed of boiled brown rice.

BROCCOLI DELIGHT

(SERVES 4)

1 lb (400g) frozen broccoli florets
Flan case
2 oz (50g) oats
2 oz (50g) wholewheat flour
1 teaspoon baking powder
1 teaspoon dried oregano
1 clove garlic, crushed
salt and pepper
2 egg whites
3 fl oz (75ml) skimmed milk
Topping
3 oz (75g) low-fat cheddar cheese
3 fl oz (75ml) skimmed milk
2 egg whites
1 small onion, finely chopped
1 clove garlic, crushed
salt and pepper to taste

Preheat oven at 180°C, 350°F, or Gas Mark 5. Very lightly grease, or spray with non-stick cooking spray, an 8-inch (20cm) baking tin.

Cook broccoli until just soft. Drain well.

To prepare flan case
In a large bowl combine the oats, flour, baking powder, oregano, garlic, salt and pepper. Mix well. In a separate small bowl, mix the egg whites and milk together and beat until well blended. Add this to the dry mixture, mixing until all the ingredients are moistened. Spread this mixture evenly in the prepared baking tin.

Place the drained broccoli on top of the crust and press down firmly with the back of a spoon so that it fits well into the flan case.

To prepare topping
Grate the cheese and sprinkle it over the broccoli.

Combine all the remaining ingredients in a blender or food processor and blend until smooth. Pour over the broccoli and cheese.

Bake uncovered for 30 minutes in the preheated oven. Cut into squares and serve hot.

BROCCOLI GRATINE WITH CHEESE AND CANNELLINI TOPPING

(See page 86)

CAULIFLOWER AND COURGETTE BAKE

(SERVES 4)

2 onions
1 small to medium cauliflower
12 oz (300g) courgettes
1 egg
2½ oz (62.5g) fromage frais or yogurt
2 teaspoons cornflour
½ teaspoon French mustard
pepper and salt
4 oz (100g) low-fat cheddar cheese
1–2 oz (25–50g) wholemeal breadcrumbs
2–3 teaspoons Parmesan cheese (optional)

Peel and slice the onions. Break the cauliflower into florets and thickly slice the courgettes.

Cook the onions in boiling salted water until they are almost tender. In another pan of boiling salted water, blanch the cauliflower florets for 5 minutes, then add the courgettes and cook for a further 2 minutes. Drain and chill under cold running water until the vegetables are cold. Drain well again and place in an oven-proof dish.

Beat the egg well and mix with the fromage frais or yogurt, cornflour and mustard. Season with salt and pepper. Beat well until smooth.

Dice the cheddar cheese and add to the fromage frais mixture. Pour over the vegetables. Sprinkle the breadcrumbs over the top with the Parmesan cheese, if used.

Bake in a preheated oven at 190°C, 375°F, or Gas Mark 5 for about 25 minutes.

CHICKPEA AND FENNEL CASSEROLE

(SERVES 2)

1 clove garlic
6 oz (150g) celery
6 oz (150g) whole green beans
1 dessertspoon fennel seeds
2 tablespoons mint, chopped
3 oz (75g) cooked chickpeas
1 oz (25g) bulgar wheat
½ pint (250ml) vegetable stock
2 tablespoons soy sauce
salt and freshly ground black pepper

Crush the garlic, dice the celery and chop the green beans. Crush the fennel seeds.

Cook the chickpeas, bulgar wheat, celery, fennel and garlic gently in a little stock for about 5 minutes. Add the remaining ingredients, excluding the mint, and simmer for 20 minutes.

Serve with fresh mint and unlimited vegetables.

COTTAGE PIE

(SERVES 4)

1½ lbs (600g) potatoes
2 onions
12 oz (300g) reconstituted TVP mince – use 4 oz (100g) dry TVP and 8 fl oz (200ml) water
3 tablespoons flour
1 tablespoon tomato purée
¾ pint (375ml) water
3 fl oz (75ml) skimmed milk
1 oz (25g) low-fat cheddar cheese

Peel the potatoes and boil for 15–20 minutes until cooked. Meanwhile, finely chop the onions and dry-fry them until softened in a non-stick frying pan. Stir in the reconstituted TVP, flour and tomato purée until thoroughly mixed. Add the water, stir well and slowly bring to the boil. Simmer for 3 minutes. Place in an ovenproof dish.

Add the milk to the potato and mash until smooth. Season to taste. Place into a piping bag fitted with a vegetable star nozzle. Pipe the potatoes over the savoury mixture. Sprinkle with the cheese and grill until lightly browned.

Serve hot.

CREAMY HORSERADISH AND WATERCRESS CRUMBLE

(See page 86)

DUO OF COURGETTES AND FLAGEOLETS EN SALADE

(See page 82)

FRESH TAGLIATELLE WITH BLUE CHEESE SAUCE

(See page 81)

HEARTY HOTPOT

(SERVES 4)

1 onion
4 tomatoes
6 oz (150g) carrots
4 oz (100g) swede
4 oz (100g) parsnips
12 oz (300g) potatoes
6 oz (150g) Brussels sprouts
4 oz (100g) tinned blackeyed beans
¾ pint (375ml) vegetable stock
2 bay leaves
1 teaspoon caraway seeds
3 tablespoons red wine
2 teaspoons soy sauce
salt and black pepper

Peel and chop the onion and tomatoes. Chop the carrots, swede and parsnips. Peel and dice the potatoes. Halve the Brussels sprouts. Drain the blackeyed beans and rinse.

Dry-fry the onion in a non-stick saucepan until soft. Add 4 fl oz (100ml) vegetable stock, the carrots, bay leaves and caraway seeds and stir for a few minutes. Then add the parsnips, swede and potatoes and cook for a further 3–4 minutes. Add the Brussels sprouts, beans, tomatoes, the remainder of the stock, the red wine and soy sauce; stir well and season to taste. Cover and cook for a further 30 minutes. Remove the bay leaves and serve.

QUICK AND LOW-FAT COURGETTE LASAGNE

(See page 84)

RICE AND ALMOND PILAFF

(See page 81)

STIR-FRIED VEGETABLES WITH GINGER AND SESAME MARINADE

(See page 85)

MIXED GRAIN AND FRESH CORIANDER MEDLEY

(See page 85)

OAT AND CHEESE LOAF

(See page 95)

POTATO MADRAS

(SERVES 4)

1¼ lbs (500g) potatoes
1 large onion
8 oz (200g) sweetcorn, frozen
1 oz (25g) lentils, presoaked
14 oz (350g) tinned tomatoes
4 teaspoons curry powder
4 tablespoons vegetable stock
salt and pepper
4 oz (100g) low-fat natural yogurt
¼ cucumber

Peel the potatoes and onion. Dice the potatoes into small pieces and slice the onion. Dry-fry the potatoes and onion in a non-stick frying pan. Add all the remaining ingredients except the yogurt and cucumber, stir well and season. Cover and cook for 15–20 minutes, stirring occasionally.

Serve with the yogurt mixed with chopped cucumber.

SWEETCORN AND POTATO FRITTERS

(SERVES 2)

8 oz (200g) potatoes
8 oz (200g) sweetcorn
1 egg white
2 tablespoons fresh chopped parsley
1 teaspoon prepared mustard

Boil the potatoes for 15–20 minutes until cooked. Mash well until smooth. Boil the sweetcorn until cooked and mix with the mashed potatoes.

Whisk the egg white until it forms soft peaks and stir into the mixture, then add the parsley and mustard.

Wet your hands and make little cakes approximately 2¾ inches (7cm) across.

Dry-fry in a non-stick frying pan until golden brown on each side.

THREE-LAYER MILLET BAKE

(See page 84)

TIKKA LENTIL BAKE

(See page 80)

TOFU BURGERS

....

(SERVES 2)

1 clove garlic
1 onion
1 lb (400g) tofu
2 oz (50g) oats
½ teaspoon ground cumin
1 teaspoon chilli powder
salt and pepper to taste

Crush the garlic. Peel and finely chop the onion.

Preheat a non-stick frying pan. Place tofu in a large bowl and mash well with a fork. Add remaining ingredients and mix well.

Shape the mixture into 6 burgers and place in the pre-heated frying pan. Cook until the burgers are brown on both sides, turning carefully.

TOFU INDONESIAN STYLE

....

(See page 81)

TRICOLOUR PASTA RISOTTO

....

(See page 88)

VEGETABLE AND FRUIT CURRY

....

(SERVES 4)

1 medium-sized onion
1 large clove garlic
1–2 green chillis (according to taste)
1-inch (2.5cm) piece green ginger
½ pint (250ml) vegetable stock
2 teaspoons garam masala
1 teaspoon ground coriander
1 teaspoon ground cumin
8 oz (200g) green beans
12 oz (300g) cauliflower florets
1 red pepper
salt
2 bananas

Prepare the ingredients: peel and chop the onion and crush the garlic. Deseed and finely chop the chillis and peel and finely grate the ginger.

Using a non-stick frying pan, dry-fry the chopped onion, garlic, chillis and ginger for 5 minutes on a gentle heat and cover the pan with a lid. Add a little of the vegetable stock if it is too dry.

When the onions are soft, add 2 fl oz (50ml) of the vegetable stock and then sprinkle in the spices and cook for a further minute, stirring all the while.

Trim the beans and cut into 1-inch (2.5cm) lengths. Break the cauliflower into small florets. Deseed and finely chop the red pepper. Add the beans, cauliflower and pepper to the pan and cook over a moderate heat for 2–3 minutes, stirring continually. Pour in the remaining vegetable stock and season with salt. Cover the pan and cook gently for 10 minutes.

Peel and slice the bananas and add to the pan. Cook for a further 10 minutes or until the vegetables are tender.

Serve with boiled brown rice, and yogurt mixed with chopped cucumber and a little mint sauce.

VEGETABLE CURRY

....

(SERVES 4)

3 oz (75g) [dry weight] soya chunks or chopped tofu, or tinned vegetable protein
1 eating apple
1 medium onion
15 oz (375g) tinned tomatoes
1 bay leaf
2 teaspoons oil-free sweet pickle or Branston pickle
1 teaspoon tomato purée
1 tablespoon curry powder

Soak the soya chunks in 2 cups of boiling water for 10 minutes. Drain.

Meanwhile, peel and chop the apple and onion. Place the soya chunks and all other ingredients in a saucepan and bring to the boil. Cover the saucepan and simmer for about 1 hour, stirring occasionally. If the mixture is too thin, remove the lid and cook on a slightly higher heat until the sauce reduces and thickens.

Serve on a bed of boiled brown rice.

VEGETABLE MIREPOIX IN FILO OVERCOAT

(See page 82)

VEGETABLE KEBABS

(SERVES 2)

1 green pepper
1 red pepper
1 large Spanish onion or 6 oz (150g) small button onions
8 oz (200g) button mushrooms
4 courgettes
1 lb (400g) average-sized fresh tomatoes
1 teaspoon thyme
cayenne pepper

Deseed the green and red peppers and chop into ¾-inch (1.8cm) squares. Peel the Spanish onion and cut into large pieces (if using the button onions just peel them). Wash and trim the mushrooms. Coarsely slice the courgettes. Halve the tomatoes.

Thread vegetable pieces alternately on four skewers to make four kebabs.

Cover a baking sheet with foil and place the kebabs on the foil, sprinkling each kebab with thyme. Wrap the foil around the kebabs to make a parcel and cook in a preheated oven at 180°C, 350°F, or Gas Mark 4 for 35 minutes.

Remove from oven. Place on a bed of hot sweetcorn and boiled rice and sprinkle with cayenne pepper to taste. Return to the oven for 1 minute.

VEGETABLE PILAFF

(SERVES 4)

1½ pints (750ml) water
2 vegetable stock cubes
10 oz (250g) [dry weight] brown rice
4 oz (100g) sweetcorn
4 oz (100g) frozen or tinned peas
1 large onion
1 red pepper
1 wineglass white wine
4 oz (100g) red kidney beans

In a large saucepan bring the water to the boil, add the stock cubes and then the brown rice. Bring back to the boil and simmer until soft but not overcooked.

In a small saucepan add the sweetcorn and peas to ½ pint (250ml) water. Bring to the boil and remove from the heat.

Peel and finely chop the onion. Wash and deseed the pepper and chop it finely. Preheat a non-stick frying pan and cook the onion until it begins to turn brown. Then add the chopped pepper and cook until both are soft. Add the white wine and the beans, peas and sweetcorn. Simmer on a very low heat until the wine has been reduced and absorbed by the vegetables. Keep it warm.

Add the cooked rice to the vegetables in the frying pan and mix well. Serve immediately on a preheated serving plate.

NB If the rice becomes too dry during cooking, add more water. If all the stock has not been absorbed at the end of cooking, drain the rice through a colander. However, do not rinse the cooked rice as this will remove the vegetable flavouring from the stock cubes.

VEGETARIAN GOULASH

(SERVES 2)

3 oz (75g) soya chunks
1 large onion
3 oz (75g) carrots
1 red pepper
3 oz (75g) potatoes
15 oz (375g) tinned tomatoes
½ pint (250ml) vegetable
stock
2 bay leaves
2 teaspoons paprika
3 tablespoons low-fat natural
yogurt
salt and black pepper to taste

Soak the soya chunks in 2 cupfuls of boiling water for 10 minutes and drain.

Meanwhile, peel and chop the onion. Slice the carrots and deseed and chop the red pepper. Peel the potatoes and cut into small chunks.

Place all the ingredients except the yogurt in a saucepan. Bring to the boil, cover and simmer for about 1 hour. Stir in the yogurt and season to taste.

VEGETARIAN LOAF

(SERVES 4)

1 lb (400g) medium tofu
8 fl oz (200ml) Bolognese
sauce (low-fat, vegetarian
brand)
1 medium onion, peeled and
finely chopped
1 green pepper, deseeded and
chopped
1 clove garlic, crushed
1 teaspoon dried oregano
½ teaspoon dried basil
1 oz (25g) oats
1 oz (25g) wholewheat flour
salt and pepper

Very lightly oil or spray with a non-stick spray a 4 × 8 inch (10 × 20cm) tin.

Rinse and drain the tofu and place it in a large bowl with half the Bolognese sauce. Add the chopped onion, pepper and spices and mash well with a fork. Add the oats, wholewheat flour, seasoning and mix well. Press the mixture into the prepared tin and press down firmly. Bake for 45 minutes in a preheated oven at 180°C, 350°F, or Gas Mark 5.

Heat the remaining sauce ready to serve with the loaf, which should be allowed to stand for 5 minutes before inverting on to a serving dish.

Serve with the hot sauce and unlimited vegetables.

VEGETABLE RISOTTO

(SERVES 4)

1 green pepper
1 red pepper
1 large onion
2 oz (50g) mushrooms
6 oz (150g) [dry weight]
brown rice
½ teaspoon oregano
8 oz (200g) tinned tomatoes
1 wine glass white wine
2 oz (50g) frozen peas
salt and freshly ground black
pepper

Prepare the vegetables. Deseed and finely chop the green and red peppers. Peel and chop the onion. Wash, trim and slice the mushrooms.

Simmer the rice in salted water until it is half-cooked. Bring a fresh pint of water to boil in another saucepan and add the half-cooked rice.

Meanwhile, dry-fry the onion and peppers in a non-stick frying pan, together with the oregano. When the onion is soft and brown in colour, add the tinned tomatoes, mushrooms, glass of wine and the frozen peas and cook for a few more minutes. When the rice is almost cooked, drain it and stir it into the vegetable mixture. Add salt and pepper to taste.

Serve immediately.

SIDE DISHES: SALADS AND VEGETABLES

CHILLI SALAD

(See page 91)

CHINESE APPLE SALAD

(See page 92)

COLESLAW

(SERVES 4)

2 large carrots
½ lb (200g) white cabbage
1 Spanish onion
4 oz (100g) reduced-oil salad
dressing (any brand)

Wash the carrots and cabbage, then grate them; peel and finely chop the onion. Mix together in a bowl with the reduced-oil salad dressing.

Keep chilled and eat within 2 days.

COURGETTE AND TOMATO SALAD

(See page 92)

SPINACH AND MUSHROOM SALAD

(SERVES 6–8)

4 oz (100g) young small spinach leaves
4 oz (100g) lambs lettuce
½ bunch watercress
4 spring onions
4 oz (100g) button mushrooms
4 tomatoes
oil-free vinaigrette
nasturtium or borage flowers (optional)

Wash the spinach and lambs lettuce well. Remove any stalks from the spinach. Wash the watercress and break into small sprigs. Trim and thinly slice the spring onions. Wipe and thinly slice the mushrooms. Peel and deseed the tomatoes and cut the flesh into strips.

Mix all the salad ingredients together in a large bowl. Toss in oil-free vinaigrette just before serving and, if desired, garnish the salad with nasturtium or borage flowers.

NB This salad may be used as an accompaniment to other dishes or served on its own with hot or cold meat, poultry or fish.

WALDORF SALAD

(See page 99)

MINTY MELON AND YOGURT SALAD

(See page 98)

CUCUMBER AND STRAWBERRY SALAD

(SERVES 4–6)

This is delicious served with 2 oz (50g) of cold salmon or 2 oz (50g) of cold trout per person.

1 small cucumber
6–8 oz (150–200g) strawberries
1 tablespoon white wine vinegar
salt and black pepper

Peel the cucumber and slice thinly. Slice the strawberries from top to bottom. Arrange the cucumber and strawberry slices in alternate rings on a plate. Sprinkle the vinegar over and season.

CREAMED POTATOES

Boil potatoes for 15–20 minutes until thoroughly

cooked. Drain and mash potatoes well, adding 3 tablespoons low-fat natural yogurt, plus salt and pepper to taste. Add skimmed milk from allowance as necessary.

DRY-ROAST POTATOES

(SERVES 3)

1 lb (400g) medium-sized potatoes
salt

Peel potatoes, then blanch them by plunging them into cold, salted water and bringing to the boil.

Drain thoroughly, then lightly scratch the surface of each potato with a fork, and sprinkle lightly with salt. Place on a non-stick baking tray, without fat, in a moderate oven (200°C, 400°F, or Gas Mark 6) for about 1–1½ hours.

JACKET POTATOES

1 medium-sized potato per person

Choose even-sized potatoes, scrub them well and make a single cut along each top. Roll them in salt and bake in the oven at 190°C, 375°F, or Gas Mark 5 for 1½ hours (or until they give when pressed). Make cross-cuts on top of each potato and squeeze to enlarge cuts. Add filling of your choice. Serve at once.

LYONNAISE POTATOES

(SERVES 2–4)

1 lb (400g) potatoes
2 large Spanish onions
garlic granules
¼–½ pint (125–250ml) skimmed milk
chopped parsley

Scrub (but don't peel) the potatoes. Peel the onions and slice the onions and potatoes. Place in layers in a casserole dish, sprinkling a few garlic granules between layers. Pour over enough skimmed milk almost to reach the top layer of the vegetables. Cover and cook in a moderately hot oven (200°C, 400°F, or Gas Mark 6) for 45 minutes to 1 hour or until tender. Garnish with chopped parsley and serve hot.

OVEN CHIPS

(SERVES 4)

2–3 large potatoes
1 teaspoon oil

Peel the potatoes and cut into chips. Blanch in boiling salted water for 5 minutes. Drain.

Meanwhile, brush a baking sheet with the oil and place in a preheated oven at 220°C, 425°F, or Gas Mark 7 for 7–10 minutes until the oil is very hot.

Spread the chips over the baking tray and turn them gently so that they are lightly coated with the oil.

Bake for 35–40 minutes (depending on the size of the chips) until they are soft in the middle and crisp on the outside. Turn them once or twice during the cooking time.

POTATO AND ONION BAKE

(SERVES 4–6)

1–1½ lbs (400–750g) old potatoes
6–8 oz (150–200g) onions
10 fl oz (250ml) vegetable or chicken stock
salt and freshly ground black pepper

Peel and thinly slice the potatoes and onions. The attachment on a food processor or mixer is ideal because the vegetables will cook more quickly if they are thinly and evenly sliced.

Bring the stock to the boil

and cook the onions in it for 3–4 minutes.

Place a layer of potatoes in the base of an ovenproof dish. Using a slotted spoon, remove the onions from the stock and place them on top of the potatoes. Cover with the remainder of the potatoes. Season each layer lightly.

Pour the remaining stock over the potatoes, cover with a lid or aluminium foil and bake in a preheated oven at 200°C, 400°F, or Gas Mark 6 for 1-1¼ hours until the vegetables are tender. Check them once or twice while they are cooking and press them down so that the top layer is kept moist. Uncover for the last 20 minutes of the cooking time so that the potatoes turn golden-brown on top.

RATATOUILLE

....

(SERVES 4)

8 oz (200g) courgettes
2 aubergines
2 medium onions
1 large green pepper
2 cloves garlic, optional
15 oz (375g) tinned tomatoes
2 bay leaves
salt and freshly ground black pepper

Slice the courgettes and auber-

gines. Peel and slice the onions. Halve the pepper, remove core and seeds, and cut flesh into fine strips. Chop the garlic.

Place the tinned tomatoes in a large saucepan and add all the other ingredients. Bring to the boil and skim any sediment if necessary. Cover and simmer for about 20 minutes or until all vegetables are tender. If there is too much liquid remaining, reduce this by boiling briskly for a few minutes with the lid removed.

NB Ratatouille can be used as a main course if accompanied by a 6 oz (150g) chicken joint or 8 oz (200g) [cooked weight] white fish.

LEMON GLAZED VEGETABLES

....

(SERVES 4)

1 lb (400g) small new potatoes
6 oz (150g) small new carrots
6 oz (150g) French beans
6 oz (150g) baby courgettes
4 oz (100g) mange tout
4 oz (100g) baby sweetcorn
2½ oz (62.5g) sugar
2 teaspoons French mustard
4–5 tablespoons lemon juice
grated rind of 1 lemon
1 tablespoon chopped coriander

Scrape the potatoes and carrots. Top and tail the French beans, courgettes and mange tout. Cut each bean into 2–3 pieces. If the courgettes are very small just cut into four down the length, otherwise cut in half and then quarter them lengthways.

Cook the potatoes in a pan of boiling salted water until tender.

In another pan of boiling salted water cook the carrots for about 4 minutes, then add the French beans and cook for a further 4–5 minutes. Finally, add the courgettes, mange tout and baby sweetcorn for a few minutes. Try to keep the vegetables slightly crisp.

Reserve about ¼ pint (250ml) of the mixed vegetable water and drain the rest of the vegetables. Keep hot.

Add the sugar, mustard and lemon juice to the reserved vegetable liquor and boil until syrupy.

Return the vegetables to the pan and turn carefully to coat them with the glaze. Pile into a hot serving dish and sprinkle with the grated lemon rind and the chopped coriander just before serving.

SPICY MUSHROOMS

....

(See page 99)

DESSERTS

APRICOT AND BANANA FOOL

(SERVES 4)

2 egg whites
10 drops liquid artificial
sweetener
4 bananas
2 oz (50g) dried apricots (the
no-soak variety)
8 oz (200g) low-fat Quark

Whisk the egg whites until they stand in peaks. Add the artificial sweetener.

Peel the bananas and mash them well in a bowl. Using a pair of scissors, snip the apricots into small pieces and add to the bananas. Mix with the Quark then gently fold into the beaten egg whites.

Divide into 4 individual dishes and chill until ready to serve. The fool is best served within 30 minutes.

Decorate each dish with a mint leaf or slice of lemon or lime.

BANANA AND SULTANA CAKE

(1 SERVING =
½-INCH/1.25CM SLICE)

1 lb 3 oz (475g) ripe bananas
(5 large peeled)
2 eggs
6 oz (150g) brown sugar
4 oz (100g) sultanas
8 oz (200g) self-raising flour

Mash bananas and add eggs, sugar and sultanas. Mix well, then stir in the flour. Place in a lined 2-lb (800g) loaf tin or cake tin.

Bake for 1¼ hours in a preheated oven at 180°C, 350°F, or Gas Mark 4. Store in an airtight tin for 24 hours before serving. Suitable for freezing.

This can be an economical recipe as very ripe bananas can often be purchased cheaply. Because of the number of portions that can be served from this loaf, the egg content need not be included in your allowance of 2 eggs per week.

CHEESE AND APRICOT PEARS

(See page 90)

FRUIT BRULEE

(SERVES 4)

Any assortment of fruit can be used for this sweet. Oranges, grapes and apples form a good base; pears, plums, raspberries, strawberries and redcurrants all provide a contrast in flavour and texture. Even in winter a few frozen raspberries can be used, but frozen strawberries are not recommended as they are too moist.

1 lb (400g) prepared fruit
1–2 tablespoons lemon juice
1 lb (400g) low-fat fromage
frais or yogurt
4–5 tablespoons demerara or
palm sugar

Using a small serrated knife, peel the oranges and cut out the segments. Wash the grapes, cut them in half and remove the pips. Peel, core and dice apples and pears. Toss them in lemon juice. Remove the stones from plums and cut into pieces. Wash and pick over raspberries, strawberries and redcurrants. Drain all the fruit well so that it is quite dry. Place the fruit in a heatproof dish and chill.

Preheat the grill until it is very hot. Just before you place the dish under the grill, spread the fromage frais or yogurt

---

over the fruit and sprinkle the sugar over the top. (It is important that this is done immediately before grilling, otherwise the sugar melts and does not caramelise.) Place the dish as high under the grill as possible and watch it all the time to see that it caramelises evenly. Turn the dish, if necessary, and take care that the sugar doesn't burn.

Allow to cool, then chill before serving.

GINGER SORBET

(SERVES 4)

16 oz (400g) stem ginger in ginger wine
4 tablespoons lemon juice
4 egg whites
2 honeydew melons (optional)

Place the ginger together with the wine in a food processor or blender and liquidise until smooth. Add the lemon juice.

Place the mixture in a shallow container in the deep freeze or freezing compartment of the refrigerator. When the mixture has formed ice crystals but is not solidly frozen, remove from the freezer and blend again.

In a large bowl whisk the egg whites until standing in firm peaks. Gently fold the blended ginger mixture into the egg whites. Place the mixture in a plastic container and re-freeze until needed.

Remove from the freezer and place in the refrigerator for 30 minutes before serving. This allows the sorbet to soften slightly so that it will be easier to serve.

Serve scoops of sorbet with chopped melon flesh or serve each portion on top of half a melon that has had all the seeds removed. Alternatively, serve the sorbet on its own.

GOOSEBERRY FOOL

(SERVES 4)

1 lb (400g) gooseberries
2–3 oz (50–75g) sugar or liquid artificial sweetener to taste
green food colouring (optional)
2 meringue shells
12–16 oz (300–400g) low-fat fromage frais
4 small sprigs mint

Top and tail the gooseberries and place in a pan with the sugar if used and 4–5 tablespoons of water. If using artificial sweetener, add after the fruit is cooked. Place over a low heat and cook gently until the fruit is barely soft. Remove and reserve a few whole gooseberries for decoration and cook the rest until they are soft.

Purée in a food processor or liquidiser. Rub through a sieve to remove the seeds and, if you wish, add a little green colouring. Cover and chill in the refrigerator.

Break the meringues into pieces and fold into the gooseberry purée. Layer the gooseberry mixture and fromage frais in tall glasses, ending with a layer of fromage frais. Decorate with the reserved gooseberries and sprigs of mint. Refrigerate until required.

HOT CHERRIES

(SERVES 4)

15 oz (375g) canned black cherries
3 fl oz (75ml) cherry brandy (optional)
2 teaspoons arrowroot
4 oz (100g) ice cream (non-Cornish variety)

Strain the cherries, reserving juice. Heat the cherry juice in a pan, add cherry brandy if desired, and thicken with enough slaked arrowroot (approximately 2 teaspoons mixed with water) to make a syrup. Stir in the cherries and pour over 1 oz (25g) ice cream per person.

Serve immediately.

KIM'S CAKE

....

(1 SERVING =
½-INCH/1.25CM SLICE)

1 lb (400g) dried mixed fruit
1 mug hot black tea
1 mug soft brown sugar
2 mugs self-raising flour
1 beaten egg

Soak the dried fruit overnight in the tea. The next day, mix all ingredients (including the tea) together, then place into a 2-lb (800g) loaf tin or round cake tin. Bake for 2 hours at 160°C, 325°F, or Gas Mark 3.

To make into a birthday-type fruit cake, add some cherries to the dried fruit.

This cake can be frozen.

LOW-FAT RICE PUDDING

....

(SERVES 4)

1 pint (500ml) skimmed milk
1 oz (25g) pudding rice
artificial sweetener to taste
(approximately 20 saccharin
tablets or 20 drops of liquid
sweetener)
pinch of nutmeg (optional)

Place all ingredients except nutmeg in an ovenproof dish. Sprinkle the nutmeg over the top. Cook in the oven for 2–2½ hours at 150°C, 300°F, Gas Mark 2. If the pudding is still sloppy 30–40 minutes before it is to be eaten, raise the oven temperature to 160°C, 325°F, or Gas Mark 3.

Serve hot or cold. If you intend to serve cold, remove from oven while still very moist as it will become stiffer and drier when cool.

MANGO AND STRAWBERRY BOMBE

....

(SERVES 4)

2 large fresh mangoes or 14 oz
(350g) tinned sliced mangoes
15 oz (375g) low-fat natural
yogurt
4 oz (100g) Quark or other
low-fat soft cheese
8 oz (200g) strawberries
1–2 tablespoons lemon juice
1–2 tablespoons clear honey
2 tablespoons strawberry
liqueur or Kirsch (optional)
few extra small strawberries
for decoration

Set the freezer to fast freeze and chill a 2-pint (1 litre) pudding basin.

Peel the fresh mangoes and cut out the stones. If using tinned mangoes, drain well. Cut the mango flesh into large pieces.

Purée about three-quarters of the mangoes in a food processor or liquidiser with 10 oz (250g) yogurt. Place in an electric sorbet maker or in a plastic container with a lid and freeze for 2–3 hours until almost solid.

In the meantime, purée the remainder of the mangoes and yogurt with the Quark, 6 oz (150g) of the strawberries, 1 tablespoon lemon juice, 1 tablespoon honey and the liqueur, if used, in a food processor or liquidiser until smooth. Taste and add more lemon juice and/or honey if necessary. Place in another container with a lid and freeze as before for 2–3 hours.

If the first mixture has been frozen in a plastic container, break down the ice crystals when it is almost frozen, using a food processor or an electric hand whisk. The crystals will not form if an electric sorbet maker is used.

Place the first mixture in the chilled pudding basin and, using a large spoon, mould the ice so that it is about 1 inch (2.5cm) thick around the sides and base of the basin. If the mixture is rather soft, fill the

Right: Mango and Strawberry Bombe

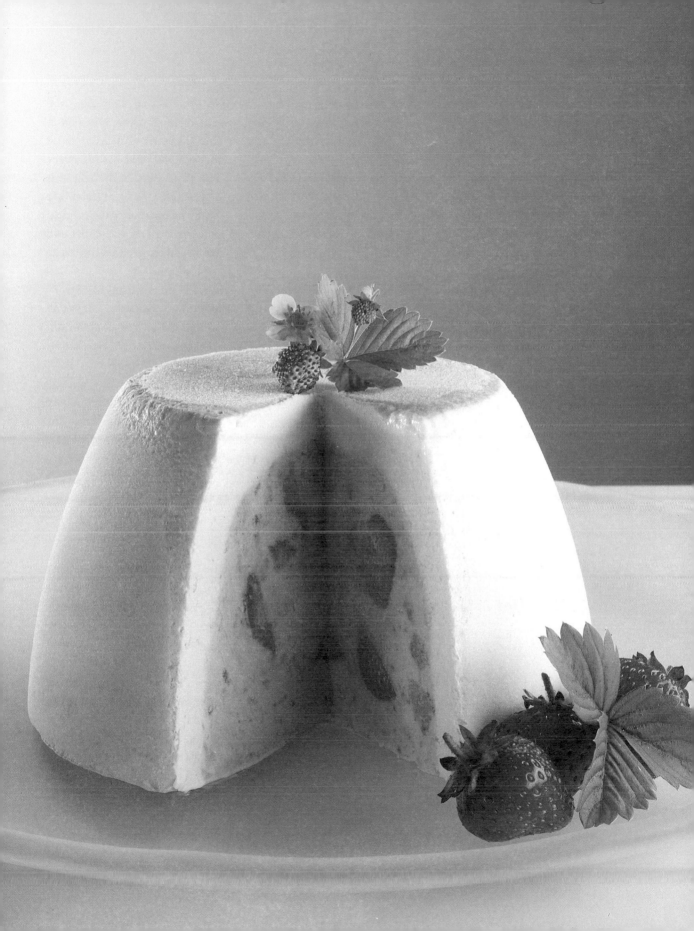

centre of the mould with a small pudding basin to keep it in place. Return it to the freezer.

Break down the crystals in the second mixture in the same way. Cut the remaining strawberries into pieces and fold into the mixture.

Remove the small basin, if used, from the ice mould. If this is firmly embedded, fill the small basin with hot water and remove immediately.

Fill the centre of the mould with the strawberry ice. Smooth over the top, cover and freeze until solid.

To serve, remove from the freezer 10–15 minutes before it is required. Dip the basin quickly into hot water and turn out on to a serving plate. Decorate with a few small strawberries.

MELON SUNDAE

(SERVES 1)

16 oz (400g) melon flesh
10 oz (250g) low-fat yogurt, any flavour, or low-fat fromage frais
8 oz (200g) green grapes

Finely chop the melon flesh and place in tall glasses. Spoon sufficient yogurt over to cover the melon. Wash, halve and seed the grapes. Divide them equally between the glasses (reserving 4 halves for decoration) and place on top of the yogurt. Add more yogurt or fromage frais on top and keep chilled until ready to serve. Decorate with 1 half-grape on top of each glass.

ORANGES GRAND MARNIER AND YOGURT SAUCE

(SERVES 4)

1 wineglass medium to sweet white wine or fresh orange juice
1 sherry glass of Grand Marnier liqueur
1 tablespoon demerara sugar or liquid artificial sweetener, if preferred
6 oranges
For the sauce
8 oz (200g) low-fat natural yogurt
2 tablespoons Grand Marnier

Heat white wine or orange juice with the liqueur in a saucepan. Add the sugar, bring to the boil and simmer until the sugar is dissolved. Allow to cool. Add liquid artificial sweetener, if used.

Carefully peel the oranges with a sharp knife to remove all pith. This can be done by slicing the peel across the top of the orange and then using the flat end of the orange as a base. Cut strips of peel away from the top downwards with a very sharp knife so that the orange is completely free from the white membranes of the pith. Squeeze the peel to extract any juice and pour this into the wine mixture.

Slice the oranges across to form round slices of equal size and place in the cool liquid. Allow to stand in a refrigerator for at least 12 hours.

Just before serving, mix the yogurt with 2 tablespoons of Grand Marnier and serve this sauce separately.

PEACH BRULEE

(SERVES 1)

3 oz (75g) tinned peaches in natural juice
3 oz (75g) low-fat fromage frais or yogurt
1 tablespoon demerara sugar

Drain the peaches and place in a ramekin dish. Spoon the fromage frais or yogurt over the fruit and sprinkle the demerara sugar on top. Immediately place under a preheated hot grill, and watch it all the time until the sugar caramelises.

Serve immediately.

PEARS IN MERINGUE

(SERVES 6)

6 ripe dessert pears, peeled
but left whole
10 fl oz (250ml) apple juice
3 egg whites
6 oz (150g) caster sugar

Cook the pears in the apple juice until just tender. Cut a slice off the bottom of each pear to enable them to sit in a dish without falling over. Place them, well spaced out, in an ovenproof dish.

Whisk the egg whites in a large and completely grease-free bowl, preferably with a balloon whisk or rotary beater, as these make more volume than an electric whisk.

When the egg whites are firm and stand in peaks, whisk in 1 tablespoon of caster sugar for 1 minute. Fold in the remainder of the sugar with a metal spoon, cutting the egg whites rather than mixing them.

Place the egg white and sugar mixture into a large piping bag with a metal nozzle (any pattern) and pipe a pyramid around each pear, starting from the base and working upwards. Place in a moderate oven at 160°C, 325°F, or Gas Mark 3, and cook until firm and golden.

Serve hot or cold.

PEARS IN RED WINE

(SERVES 4)

2 wineglasses red wine
2 fl oz (50ml) water
2 oz (50g) brown sugar
½ level teaspoon cinnamon or
ground ginger
6 ripe pears, peeled but left
whole

Combine wine, water, sugar and spice in a large saucepan, and bring to the boil. Add the pears to the pan and simmer for 10–15 minutes, turning the pears carefully from time to time to ensure even colouring.

Serve hot or cold.

PINEAPPLE, PEACH AND STRAWBERRY DESSERT

(SERVES 4–6)

1 small pineapple or 16 oz
(400g) tinned pineapple pieces
in natural juice
2 large peaches
2 tablespoons lemon juice
4 oz (100g) white seedless
grapes or 2 kiwifruit
8 oz (200g) strawberries
6 oz (150g) low-fat natural
yogurt
2 tablespoons honey
¼ teaspoon ground cinnamon

Cut the fresh pineapple in half and, using a grapefruit knife, cut out the flesh; or, if you prefer, cut the skin from the pineapple and then cut it in half. Remove the hard centre core and cut the flesh into pieces. If using tinned fruit, drain well.

Pour boiling water over the peaches and leave for 2–3 minutes. Drain and place in cold water to cool. Remove the skins and the stones and dice the flesh. Toss in the lemon juice.

Remove the stalks from the grapes or peel and slice the kiwifruit. Hull and halve the strawberries. Reserve a few grapes (or slices of kiwifruit) and a few strawberries for decoration.

Mix the yogurt, honey and cinnamon together. Add the fruit and mix well. Place in a large bowl or individual glasses. Decorate with the reserved fruit. Chill until required.

RASPBERRY FLUFF

(SERVES 4)

8 oz (200g) fresh or frozen
raspberries
1 egg white, optional
1 lb (400g) low-fat fromage
frais or low-fat yogurt
caster sugar (optional)

Wash the fresh raspberries and drain well. Reserve a few for decoration and mash the rest slightly with a fork.

Whisk the egg white in a clean dry bowl until it stands in stiff peaks. Using a metal spoon or spatula, carefully fold into the fromage frais.

Layer the fromage frais and raspberries in four tall glasses, ending with a layer of fromage frais.

Decorate the top with a few whole raspberries. Refrigerate until required and serve with caster sugar if you wish.

If you prefer to avoid the use of uncooked egg whites, omit them and just layer the fromage frais and raspberries.

RASPBERRY MOUSSE

(SERVES 4)

8 oz (200g) fresh or frozen raspberries or 7 oz (175g) tinned raspberries in natural juice
4 oz (100g) natural apple juice
approximately 15 drops liquid artificial sweetener
1 teaspoon gelatine
2 egg whites
4 teaspoons raspberry yogurt
12 fresh raspberries, to decorate

Place raspberries and apple juice in a liquidiser and blend until smooth. If using tinned raspberries, drain well. Strain through a sieve into a basin. Add liquid sweetener to taste.

Dissolve gelatine in 3 teaspoons of water in a cup over very hot water. Add to raspberry purée and stir well.

Whisk egg whites until they form peaks. Fold into purée.

Pour mixture into tall sundae glasses or a serving dish. Decorate with a teaspoon of raspberry yogurt and 3 fresh raspberries per person just before serving.

RASPBERRY YOGURT DELIGHT

(SERVES 4)

2 teaspoons gelatine
1 pint (500ml) low-fat raspberry yogurt
8 oz (200g) raspberries
2–3 tablespoons low-fat natural fromage frais or yogurt

Sprinkle the gelatine on to 2 tablespoons of cold water in a bowl. Leave for 4–5 minutes until soft, then stand the bowl over hot water and stir until the gelatine has dissolved. Stir the gelatine into the yogurt.

Stir 6 oz (150g) of the raspberries into the yogurt and leave until the mixture is on the point of setting. Stir gently to ensure that the raspberries are suspended in the yogurt jelly. Pour into individual glasses and chill until set. Decorate the top of each one with a little fromage frais or yogurt and the remaining raspberries.

NB This sweet can also be made with strawberries. In this case, slice the strawberries before placing into the jelly mixture.

MERINGUE BISCUITS

(MAKES APPROXIMATELY 30 BISCUITS)

4 egg whites
8 oz (200g) caster sugar

Whisk the egg whites until they stand in stiff peaks. Add 1 oz (25g) of the caster sugar and continue whisking for 1 minute. Fold in the remaining caster sugar.

Place the meringue mixture in a large piping bag with a large nozzle (any pattern nozzle will do). Gently pipe the egg whites into small pyramids on to a non-stick baking sheet. Place in a cool oven (150°C, 300°F, or Gas Mark 2) for approximately 2 hours or until crisp and beige in colour. The meringues should easily come away from the baking sheet. If they don't, gently prise them off with a sharp, pliable knife. Meringues may be stored in an airtight container for up to 2 weeks.

RED FRUIT SALAD

....

(SERVES 6)

12 oz (300g) strawberries
8 oz (200g) raspberries
8 oz (200g) redcurrants
4 oz (100g) blackcurrants
4 oz (100g) dark red cherries
4 oz (100g) dark red plums
2–3 tablespoons sugar or
artificial sweetener to taste
2 teaspoons arrowroot
2 tablespoons Kirsch, optional
8 oz (200g) low-fat fromage
frais or low-fat natural yogurt
meringue fingers

Hull the strawberries and raspberries. Remove the stalks from the other fruits. Stone the cherries if desired and remove the stones from the plums. Cut the plums into ½-inch (1.25cm) dice.

Place the redcurrants and blackcurrants in a pan with ½ pint (250ml) water and simmer gently for 4–5 minutes until the fruit is only just tender and holds its shape. Add sugar or sweetener to taste. Mix the arrowroot with a little water and add to the pan. Bring to the boil, stirring all the time. Add the remainder of the fruit, and the Kirsch, if used, and allow to cool slightly.

Pour into a large bowl or individual bowls. Chill until required. Serve with fromage frais or yogurt, and meringue fingers.

STRAWBERRY SORBET

....

(SERVES 4)

1 lb (400g) strawberries
2 large egg whites
liquid artificial sweetener to
taste (optional)
additional fresh strawberries,
to serve

Wash and hull the strawberries and place them in a large saucepan with very little water (just enough to prevent the strawberries sticking to the pan). Cover with a lid and simmer gently on a low heat until the fruit becomes soft and the juice runs. Place the mixture in a food processor and liquidise or, alternatively, rub the fruit through a sieve using a wooden spoon.

Allow to cool and place the purée in a shallow container. Cover with cling film or foil and place in the freezer or the deep-freeze compartment of the refrigerator until the purée begins to set and crystallise. Remove the mixture from the freezer and stir it to form a soft crystallised consistency.

Whisk the two egg whites until stiff and standing in peaks. Fold into the semi-frozen purée to give a marbled effect. Immediately return the mixture to the freezer and freeze until firm. Store in the freezer until required.

Remove from the freezer and place in the refrigerator 30 minutes before serving. Serve with fresh strawberries.

SUMMER PUDDING

....

(SERVES 6)

Any selection of summer fruits can be used. Raspberries, redcurrants and blackcurrants are ideal, but take care not to use more than approximately 6 oz (150g) of blackcurrants or their flavour will become too dominant. Blackberries, gooseberries, red cherries, red plums and strawberries can also be used. Stone cherries and plums and cut each half of plums into 3–4 pieces. Cut large strawberries into quarters; leave small ones whole.

Use day-old bread for this

pudding. Cut it about as thick as you would for sandwiches. Baker's bread is better than sliced pre-packed bread.

8–10 thin slices of bread
1½ lbs (600g) soft fruit
4 oz (100g) sugar
low-fat fromage frais, to serve

Cut the crusts from the bread and from one slice cut a circle about 1 inch (2.5cm) wider than the base of a 1½-pint (750ml) pudding basin. Reserve 1–2 slices to cover the top and cut the remainder of the bread into wedge shapes. Place the circle of bread in the base of the basin and arrange the wedge shapes around the side, making certain that they overlap in all places. If there should be a small gap anywhere, patch it on the inside with a small piece of bread. If you prefer, just line the inside of the basin with the slices of bread, rather than wedges. You will not waste any bread this way but it will look slightly less attractive.

Prepare the fruit as described and place blackcurrants, redcurrants, blackberries, gooseberries, cherries and plums (according to the selection used) in a pan with the sugar and ¼ pint (125ml) water. Bring to the boil and simmer for 2–3 minutes. Add the raspberries and cook for a further

minute. Add strawberries, if used, and remove from the heat. It is not necessary to cook the fruit until it is soft, only until the sugar has dissolved and the juices are running from the fruit. With a slotted spoon, remove the fruit from the syrup and place in the prepared basin with sufficient syrup to moisten the bread. Reserve the remainder of the syrup. Cover the top of the basin completely with bread. Place a piece of food wrap over the pudding and put a lightly weighted saucer on top. Refrigerate overnight or for at least 6–8 hours.

Turn out the pudding carefully on to a serving dish. If any parts of the bread have not been saturated by the syrup, spoon a little of the reserved syrup over. Serve the rest separately, together with a bowl of low-fat fromage frais.

SUMMER SURPRISE

(SERVES 4)

1 small pineapple or 8 oz (200g) tinned pineapple in natural juice
8 oz (200g) small strawberries
8 oz (200g) blackcurrants, fresh or frozen
icing sugar or artificial sweetener to taste

low-fat natural fromage frais or yogurt, to serve

Cut the skin from the pineapple, cut in half and remove the hard centre core. Cut the rest of the pineapple into dice, or drain the tinned pineapple. Wash and hull the strawberries and mix with the pineapple. Place the fruit in 4 dishes.

Remove the stalks from fresh blackcurrants. Cook in a scant 5 fl oz (125ml) water until tender. Purée very lightly in a food processor or liquidiser (only enough to break down the fruit – take care not to purée the seeds). Rub the blackcurrant mixture through a sieve to remove the seeds. Add icing sugar or sweetener to taste.

Pour the blackcurrant purée over the pineapple and strawberries just before serving. Serve topped with fromage frais or yogurt.

TROPICAL FRUIT SALAD

(See recipe, page 170)

Right: Summer Pudding

144

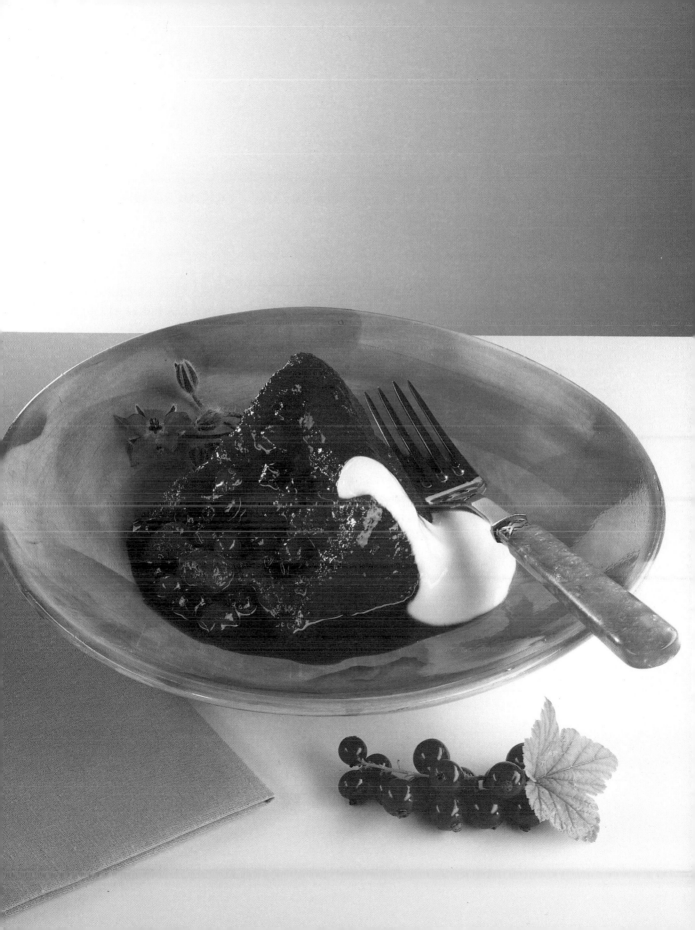

DRESSINGS

GARLIC DRESSING

1 clove garlic
5 oz (125g) low-fat natural
yogurt
1 tablespoon wine vinegar
1 tablespoon reduced-oil salad
dressing (any brand)
salt and freshly ground black
pepper

Crush the garlic and then mix
all the ingredients together.
Store in a screw-top jar in the
refrigerator and use within 2
days.

CITRUS DRESSING

4 fl oz (100ml) fresh orange
juice
2 fl oz (50ml) lemon juice
2 fl oz (50ml) wine vinegar
1 teaspoon Dijon mustard
salt and pepper

Place all the ingredients in a
clean screw-top jar and shake
well. Keep in a refrigerator and
use within 3 days.

OIL-FREE VINAIGRETTE DRESSING

3 tablespoons white wine
vinegar or cider vinegar
1 tablespoon lemon juice
½ teaspoon black pepper
½ teaspoon salt
1 teaspoon sugar
½ teaspoon French mustard
chopped herbs (thyme,
marjoram, basil or parsley)

Mix all the ingredients together. Place in a container,
seal and shake well. Taste, and
add more salt or sugar as
desired.

MARIE ROSE DRESSING

(SERVES 2)

2 tablespoons tomato ketchup
1 tablespoon reduced-oil salad
dressing (any brand)
dash Tabasco sauce
squeeze lemon juice

Mix all ingredients together
well and store in a screw-top
jar in the refrigerator until
needed.

REDUCED-OIL DRESSING

Mix 3 tablespoons reduced-oil,
low-calorie salad dressing (any
brand) with 5 oz (125g) plain
low-fat yogurt. Add salt and
pepper to taste.

Keeps in a refrigerator for up
to 2 days.

YOGURT DRESSING

5 oz (125g) natural yogurt
good squeeze lemon juice
salt and freshly ground black
pepper

Mix all the ingredients together
and use as a dressing for salad.
As a variation, add ½ teaspoon
prepared mint sauce.

MAINTAINING YOUR WEIGHT-LOSS

For those who still have weight to lose, it is important to continue with the diet plan. If you do so, you will lose further weight and inches (centimetres). However, it is essential to realise that simply just 'not eating fat' is not sufficient to enable you to lose weight. Such a principle is fine for maintenance but not for those wishing to slim down further.

As explained earlier, losing weight is comparatively easy because we have a definite plan of action to follow, the basis of which is to cut down on calories so that our body will burn away its excesses. But when we attempt to *maintain* that loss, the going can be tricky. The object is simple: we need to try to balance the energy value of the food we eat with the calories we burn up in everyday living.

The good news is that if we continue to follow a relatively low-fat diet, maintenance is actually very easy. All we need to do is increase the amount of low-fat foods to satisfy our individual appetite, but still restrict the intake of fatty foods. This is easier than we might imagine, because after three or four weeks on a low-fat diet our taste buds adapt and the taste of greasy food can become quite repulsive. By sticking to low-fat foods and increasing the amount of carbohydrates we eat we can enjoy plenty of volume of food and need never feel hungry.

Because of the feeling of wellbeing experienced by those following a well-balanced, nutritious, but very low-fat diet it may be tempting to give up fatty foods for ever. It would, however, be impossible to eat a completely fat-free diet unless we lived solely on vegetables. In any case, we do need a certain amount of fat in our daily diet, as I explained earlier (see page 21), and providing our diet is varied we will never become deficient in it. After we have reached our desired weight and size we can increase the amount of fat we consume by a small amount without experiencing any deterioration to our health or shape. Having the occasional treat, therefore, or even simply reintroducing some low-fat spread on to your bread is quite acceptable. But once you start adding fat to your diet again make sure you don't find yourself on a slippery slope, falling back into previous unhealthy eating habits. Proceed with caution!

The following lists itemise those foods which form the basis of a healthy diet that will enable you to maintain your new lower weight. You may select freely from food on the **Green** list without worrying about quantities unless it specifies 'in moderation'. You may also select occasionally from the **Amber** list, but avoid the **Red** list as much as possible. The occasional overindulgence, however, will do little damage as long as it does not lead to another one! Just remember that fat you eat equals fat on your body. Take the trouble to check the nutrition panel on every can or packet that you buy. Look for brands with the lowest amount of fat and don't be misled by the breakdown of saturated or unsaturated fats. As far as a low-fat diet is concerned it is the TOTAL fat content that matters, and that will be the highest of these figures under the FAT heading.

Keep an eye on the scales and the tape measure. If you find you are gaining a little in either direction, go back on to the diet or just cut back on your quantities. Usually we know how and when the damage was caused! If we take immediate action, the remedy can be swift. Allow yourself a margin of fluctuation of no more than 2 lbs (1kg). If you go beyond that limit, take action immediately. Don't starve yourself, simply go back to the diet plan and eat what it says. Don't be tempted to hurry things along by missing meals. You won't lose your weight any more quickly. In fact it is likely to take longer because you'll cheat and that may lead to a binge. So be sensible, be relaxed. Just follow the diet and the diet will look after you.

Eat three meals a day and eat sufficient at each meal to satisfy your appetite. Fill up on extra vegetables if necessary. Getting up from the dining table still feeling peckish could lead to nibbling the wrong snack foods, and eating between meals is a habit that should be curbed.

Try to exercise three times a week for at least 20 minutes each time, and be aware that exercise that makes you puff is helping to keep your heart fitter too. Exercise should be enjoyable, so find a way of keeping fit that is fun (see page 22). Try to PLAN your exercise, preferably with a friend, so that you keep to it, or, better still, exercise as a family.

Remember, eating should be a pleasurable experience too, and if you follow a basically low-fat formula you should still be able to eat well, look better, feel fitter and live longer. Educating our families to eat healthily is the best inheritance we can give them. And it's never too late to start.

GREEN

Most of the following foods may be eaten freely but restrict the quantities of those specified to be consumed in moderation.

Alcohol: any type, except cream liqueur, in moderation (not exceeding 21 units a week for men and 14 units a week for women)
Beans, lentils and pulses: any type
Bread: any type without fat (not fried or buttered)
Breakfast cereal: any type
Cakes: cakes made with little or no fat (e.g. Kim's Cake, Banana and Sultana Cake (see recipes, pages 138 and 136)
Cheese: cottage cheese, fromage frais, Quark (choose low-fat varieties)
Condiments: any type except tartar sauce (see also **Sauces**)
Crispbreads: rye crispbreads, Ryvita
Dressings: lemon juice; oil-free dressings, reduced-oil dressings in moderation, vinegar
Eggs: egg whites can be eaten freely; egg yolks (a maximum of 2 a week)
Fish (including shellfish): any type of white fish (e.g. cod, plaice, halibut, whiting, lemon sole), cockles, crab, lobster, mussels, oysters, prawns, salmon, shrimps, tuna in brine; mackerel in moderation
Flour: any type
Fruit: any type of fresh, frozen or tinned fruit, except ackee, avocado, coconut and olives; dried fruit in moderation
Fruit juices: apple juice, exotic fruit juices, grapefruit, grape juice, unsweetened orange and pineapple
Game: any type, roasted without fat and with all skin removed

Grains: any type (see also **Rice**)

Gravy: made with gravy powder, not granules, unless low-fat varieties

Jams, preserves and spreads: honey, jam, Marmite, Bovril, marmalade, syrup – all in moderation.

Meat: lean red meat (twice a week maximum) cooked without fat (see also **Game, Offal, Poultry**)

Meat substitutes: textured vegetable protein, vegeburgers

Milk: skimmed or semi-skimmed (silver top with cream removed can be classed as semi-skimmed)

Nuts: chestnuts only

Offal: any type in moderation, cooked without fat

Pasta: egg-free and fat-free varieties

Pickles and relishes: any type

Poultry: chicken, duck, turkey – all cooked without fat and with all skin removed

Prepared meals for slimmers: Boots, Lean Cuisine, Menu Plus, Weight Watchers ranges

Puddings: custard (made with skimmed milk), fresh fruit salad, low-fat varieties of fromage frais, fruit cooked with wine, jelly, meringues, rice pudding (made with skimmed milk), low-fat varieties of yogurt

Rice: brown rice, boiled or steamed

Sauces: apple sauce, brown sauce, cranberry sauce, horseradish, mint sauce, tomato ketchup, soy sauce, white sauces made with skimmed milk and no fat, Worcestershire sauce (see also **Condiments**)

Snacks: tropical fruit mix in moderation

Soups: clear and non-cream varieties

Soya: low-fat type

Stuffing: made with water

Sugar: any type in moderation; artificial sweeteners

Vegetables: any type (except ackee and avocado), cooked and served without fat

Yogurt: any low-fat varieties; avoid Greek yogurt

AMBER

Alcohol: Any except cream liqueur (not exceeding 21 units a week for men and 14 units a week for women, see page 28)

Bread: bread spread with low-fat spread

Cakes, biscuits and pastries: Jaffa cakes, filo pastry; savoury biscuits such as cream crackers or water biscuits

Cheese: cheese spread, Edam, Gouda, low-fat hard cheeses, low-fat soft cheese

Confectionery: fat-free types

Dressings: low-fat mayonnaise

Drinks: low-fat malted drinks such as low-fat varieties of Horlicks, Ovaltine, drinking chocolate – all made with skimmed milk; tea and coffee made with milk; yogurt drinks

Eggs and egg products: in moderation; Yorkshire pudding made with skimmed milk and cooked in a non-stick baking tin with no fat

Fats and spreads: low-fat spreads with a fat content of less than 50 per cent

Fish: bloaters, eels, fish fingers (grilled), fish in sauces (branded products), herrings, kippers (cooked without butter), rollmop herrings, sardines, sprats

Jams and preserves: lemon curd in moderation

Meat and meat products: beefburgers (grilled), corned beef, faggots, lamb chops (grilled), low-fat sausages (grilled), meat with some fat (such as streaky bacon), roast meat

Milk, cream and similar products: Dream Topping, full-fat milk, single cream, Tip-Top

Pasta: pasta made with eggs and flour but served without butter

Prepacked meals: check nutrition panel and choose the brand with the lowest fat content

Puddings: regular custard, ice cream (not Cornish varieties), pavlova, regular rice pudding, sponge flan, trifle

Sauces: sauces (sweet or savoury) made with full-fat milk but without butter, e.g. parsley sauce, white sauce

Snacks: low-fat crisps, twiglets

Soups: all branded soups and soups made without cream, fat or butter

Sugar: syrup

Vegetables: thick-cut chips, oven chips

Yogurt: creamy yogurts, Greek yogurt

RED

Alcohol: cream liqueurs

Bread: garlic bread

Cakes and biscuits: all cakes and pastries not included in other lists; all sweet biscuits; savoury biscuits containing cheese or butter

Cheese: full-fat cheeses, any kind

Confectionery: butterscotch, caramel, chocolates, fudge, toffees

Dressings: all oils, cream dressings, French dressing, mayonnaise

Drinks: cocoa and cocoa products, e.g. Ovaltine (unless low-fat variety), regular Horlicks, tea or coffee with cream

Eggs and egg products: custard tarts, egg custards, quiches, Scotch eggs, Yorkshire pudding cooked in fat

Fats and spreads: butter, dripping, lard, low-fat spreads with more than 50% fat content, margarine, margarines high in polyunsaturates, oil (all kinds), peanut butter, suet

Fish: fish in batter, fried fish, fried fishcakes, kippers in butter, fried whitebait

Fruit: avocado pears

Meat and meat products: black pudding, fatty meat, full-fat sausages, German sausage, haggis, haslet, liver sausage, meat fried in breadcrumbs, meat fried (such as fried beefburgers), meat pies, pasties, pâté (except chicken liver pâté), pork pie, salami, sausages in batter, tongue

Milk, cream and similar products: butter cream, double cream, gold top milk, Jersey milk, whipping cream

Marzipan

Nuts: all nuts except chestnuts; sunflower seeds

Pasta: pasta served with butter

Poultry: goose, skin from any poultry

Puddings: chocolate ice creams, Cornish ice creams, crème brûlée, gâteaux, pastries, pies, profiteroles with chocolate sauce, roulades, soufflés

Rice: fried rice

Sauces: cheese sauce, Hollandaise sauce, sauces made with butter and/or cream

Snacks: cheeselets and similar biscuits, regular crisps and similar fried snacks, olives, peanuts

Vegetables: ackee, avocado, thin or crinkle-cut chips, vegetables served in butter, fried or roasted with fat

PACKED LUNCH IDEAS FOR CHILDREN

Kim Hames is a 33-year-old wife and mum who works part-time as a school teacher. Kim joined my slimming and exercise class weighing 16 st 7 lbs (104.7kg). Within a year she lost 6 stone (38.1kg) by following my Complete Hip & Thigh Diet. She has now reduced her weight by almost 7 stone (44.5kg). It is Kim who supplied the recipe for the virtually fat-free Kim's Cake (see page 138). Her talent for understanding the desires of children, coupled with her knowledge of low-fat eating, prompted me to ask Kim to create ten healthy, low-fat packed lunches. I hope *your* children will enjoy Kim's creations.

TEN LOW-FAT PACKED LUNCHES

Sandwiches are probably the first things that spring to mind when we think of preparing a packed lunch, and here you'll find some suggestions for tasty sandwich fillings. Make the sandwiches *without* spreading on fat. Vary the shapes, using biscuit cutters, and introduce a theme for the day. For example, rabbit-shaped sandwiches could be accompanied by carrot sticks; or have everything round, or chip-shaped or square!

I have also included other ideas for packed lunches that are simple to achieve *without* too much preparation. I like to use up leftovers if ever there are any! Cooked pasta, for instance, could be mixed with tuna and apple for lunch. Cold pizza or cold cooked chicken are popular

favourites and so are home-made Beefburgers in a Bap (see recipe, page 154). Large cakes can be cut into fingers, or cut to fit inside paper cake cases, if your child prefers. If cooking cakes and making savoury loaves does not appeal to you, then take note of the fat and sugar content in any you buy. Try to avoid buying snack bars and crisps as a matter of routine. Use them only as 'special treats'.

Invest in a good lunch box that is large enough to hold a pot of your child's favourite yogurt.

- Tuna sandwich (spread the bread with low-fat salad cream and fill with drained tuna – canned in brine not oil – and lettuce)
- Low-fat fromage frais
- Apple pieces

- French Bread Pizza (see recipe, page 152)
- Low-fat yogurt
- Dried banana chips

- Slice of Salmon Loaf (see recipe, page 152)
- Cucumber cut into chip shapes
- Gingerbread People (see recipe, page 154)
- Satsuma

- Pitta bread filled with diced chicken, lettuce, tomato and cucumber
- Slice of Banana and Sultana Cake (see recipe, page 136)

- Crunchy Vegetable Dip (see recipe, page 152)
- Slice of Kim's Cake (see recipe, page 138)
- Low-fat yogurt

- Beefburger in Bap (see recipe, page 154)
- Apple, raisins and marshmallows – cut into pieces

- Cucumber Rings (see recipe, page 154) and crackers
- Spiced Buns (see recipe, page 154)
- Satsuma

- Wafer-thin Sandwiches (see below)
- Jam Swiss roll
- Pear

- Mashed banana and raisin sandwich
- Low-fat fromage frais
- Apple pieces

- Slice of Minced Pork Loaf (see recipe, page 154)
- Low-fat rice pudding or custard (any brand)
- Satsuma or banana

FRENCH BREAD PIZZA

Cut off a section of French stick and halve it. Spread with tomato sauce. Add ham and pineapple, or mackerel in tomato sauce. Sprinkle lightly with low-fat hard cheese. Bake in a preheated oven at 180°C, 350°F, or Gas Mark 4 for 5 minutes or until the cheese melts.

CRUNCHY VEGETABLE DIP

Cut a selection of vegetables (carrots, cucumber, celery, cauliflower and apple) into sticks. Make up the dip by mixing 1 tablespoon of smooth peanut butter with 2 tablespoons of cottage cheese. Alternatively, mix 2 tablespoons of low-fat cheese spread with 1 tablespoon of tomato purée.

SALMON LOAF

3 slices white bread made into crumbs
12 oz (300g) drained canned salmon (reserve juice)
1 oz (25g) non-fat dry milk mixed with juice from canned salmon and made up to nearly ½ pint (8 fl oz/200ml) with water
1 tablespoon dried onion flakes mixed with 1 tablespoon of water
1 teaspoon lemon juice
2 eggs, beaten
2 eggs, hard-boiled

In a large bowl mix the bread crumbs with the milk, salmon juice and water mixture. Leave for 10 minutes to soak.

In a smaller bowl mix together the salmon, onion flakes, lemon juice and beaten eggs. Add to bread mixture and mix.

Spoon half the mixture into a 1-lb (400g) loaf tin lined with parchment paper on the base.

Shell the hard-boiled eggs and place them in the centre of the salmon mixture. Cover with the remaining mixture.

Bake at 180°C, 350°F, or Gas Mark 4 for 50 minutes or until loaf is firm and browned.

Serve in slices.

WAFER-THIN SANDWICHES

Roll slices of bread with a rolling pin until very thin. Spread each slice with low-fat cheese spread and place wafer-thin ham on top. Roll up each slice to make a long sausage shape.

Wafer-thin turkey and pork, available in most large supermarket delicatessens, can also be used.

Right: Crunchy Vegetable Dip; slice of Kim's Cake

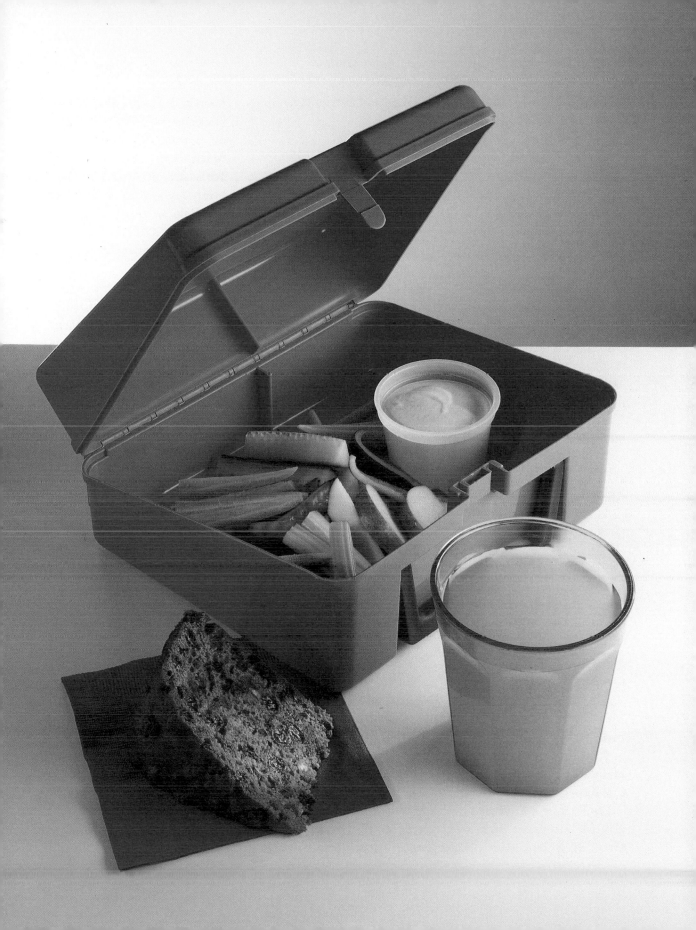

MINCED PORK LOAF

....

1½ lbs (600g) minced pork
1 onion, chopped
2 oz (50g) fresh breadcrumbs
1 tablespoon parsley
pinch curry powder
pinch garlic salt
1 egg, beaten

Mix all the ingredients together in a large bowl. Place in a non-stick 2-lb (800g) loaf tin. Place inside a larger size baking tin half-filled with water. Bake in a preheated oven at 200°C, 400°F, or Gas Mark 6 for 1½ hours. Serve cold.

BEEFBURGER IN BAP

....

(SERVES 4)

1 onion, chopped
1 lb (400g) minced beef
3 tablespoons breadcrumbs
4 tablespoons milk
4 burger buns
4 tomato slices
tomato ketchup

Mix chopped onion, minced beef, breadcrumbs and milk in a large bowl. Leave for 10 minutes and then make up mixture into 4 beefburgers.

Cook under a preheated hot grill for 5 minutes each side. Place in a bun with sliced tomato and tomato ketchup.

CUCUMBER RINGS

....

1 cucumber
3½ oz (87.5g) tinned pink salmon
2 tablespoons low-fat cheese spread
1 teaspoon tomato purée
squeeze of lemon

Cut cucumber into 8 large rings, each 1 inch (2.5cm) in length. With a teaspoon, scoop the seeds out of each ring to leave a shell ½ inch (1.25cm) thick. Mix remaining ingredients and use to fill the rings.

Serve with crunchy crackers.

SPICED BUNS

....

(MAKES 12 BUNS)

1 egg, beaten
½ pint (10 fl oz/250ml) water
1 lb (400g) self-raising flour
1 teaspoon mixed spice
3 oz (75g) sugar
2 oz (50g) margarine
8 oz (200g) mixed fruit

Put aside 1 teaspoon of beaten egg. Mix remainder of egg with all other ingredients to form a soft dough. Divide the dough into 12 pieces and place on a floured surface. Shape into buns and roll out a little. Place on a non-stick baking tray. Make deep right-angle cuts across the tops of each bun and brush over with remainder of egg. Bake in a preheated oven at 220°C, 425°F, or Gas Mark 7 until the tops are brown.

GINGERBREAD PEOPLE

....

(MAKES APPROX. 20 PEOPLE)

3 tablespoons golden syrup
2 oz (50g) margarine
4 oz (100g) sugar
10 oz (250g) self-raising flour
2 teaspoons ground ginger
4 tablespoons milk
currants and glacé cherries

Preheat the oven at 170°C, 320°F, Gas Mark 3. Warm the syrup, margarine and sugar in a pan over a low heat. Place flour and ginger into a bowl and add the syrup mixture. Pour in the milk and mix until gooey.

Roll out on a floured surface and then, using a body-shaped cutter, cut out 'people'. Use the currants for eyes and buttons, and a quarter slice of cherry for each mouth. Place on to non-stick baking trays and bake for 10–15 minutes. Remove from oven and transfer *immediately* to a cooling rack.

HOW TO ENJOY CHRISTMAS WITHOUT RUINING YOUR DIET

Each year as Christmas approaches, I have to admit to a touch of apprehension. Even if I have managed to stay on top of controlling my weight for most of the year, there is always the danger of so much damage being done over Christmas and New Year. At this special time of the year we want to treat our family to lots of goodies we wouldn't usually buy, stocking up the store cupboard in the weeks leading up to Christmas. Then on Christmas Day we proudly display a magnificent selection of delicious delicacies. But since mealtimes play such a major role in celebrating Christmas, often the chocolates, Turkish Delight and nuts remain barely touched. Then, after the festivities are over, because we can't bear to see food wasted – we eat them! And THAT is where a lot of the damage is done.

I would never expect anyone to lose weight over Christmas, and I do think we should allow ourselves lots of treats, as it is very important for the dieter to feel he or she is not missing out. I have discovered that when I have been positively saintly over Christmas, my willpower has subsequently disintegrated around New Year. I have now resolved this problem. I have found that we actually NEED to overeat at Christmas. Having a bit of a blow-out and then feeling so uncomfortable afterwards reminds us of how much better we feel when we eat sensibly. So by making a few simple changes to the way festive food is prepared, in order to minimise the damage, I am able to spoil myself, even over-indulge, so that I never feel I am going without. On this basis I can eat as much as I want on both Christmas and Boxing Day. The following day I feel so overfull that I start my Christmas Binge Corrector Diet. Any excess weight swiftly disappears and I go back to eating sensibly from then on.

None of my family is on a diet, and the first time I prepared my special Christmas lunch they all enjoyed it without having any idea that it was cooked entirely without added fat. I challenge anyone to spot the difference between the low-fat Christmas recipes included in this book and conventional recipes. In fact I believe some of them are infinitely tastier.

As well as a Christmas menu I have included ideas for some low-fat home-made sweets and cakes. In my experience, after over-indulging in low-fat foods, any excess weight swiftly burns away if remedial action is taken. On the other hand, when I eat fatty food, the weight seems to pile on twice as quickly and is very difficult to shift. Some of these recipes include foods normally banned on my low-fat diets, such as walnuts. However, as Christmas comes but once a year (and let's hope you won't eat *too* much of any one of these treats!), I have made an exception.

TEN TIPS FOR A SLIMMER CHRISTMAS

● **1** Just because the shops will be closed for a couple of days, don't buy up your local supermarket and stock up on loads of unnecessary Christmas fare, which may still be hanging around after Christmas. It only leads to temptation.

● **2** Make a plan of your menus and requirements for the holiday period and stick to it.

● **3** If you buy nuts, always buy them in their shells. You will probably get fed up with struggling with the nutcrackers after a couple of attempts. The ready-shelled packets are just too tempting. For this reason nuts in their shells are included in the **Amber** list, while ready-shelled nuts are on the **Red** list.

● **4** Eat your main Christmas meal at around 2pm. If you eat it in the evening, you will eat more during the rest of the day.

● **5** Unless everyone else in the family enjoys Christmas cake, don't have one. It is the biggest cause of the New Year downfall for slimmers who struggle to finish it before they start dieting. If you don't have a cake, you may not need to diet at all.

● **6** Open only one box of chocolates or Turkish Delight at a time – and be extremely generous in offering them around so that they disappear quickly! Try not to eat more than two chocolates a day. Any boxes that remain unopened after Christmas could be given to a local hospital where patients could do with the extra calories as they recover from their operations.

● **7** Make it a rule not to eat between mealtimes. Always leave the table feeling satisfied. Fill up on vegetables if necessary.

● **8** Have a low-calorie drink prior to each meal. This will help fill you up and make you feel satisfied more quickly. Also remember that the more alcohol you drink, the weaker your willpower becomes, so beware!

● **9** Be as active as possible. Go for walks with the dog and the children. Part of the reason we tend to gain so much weight at Christmas is because we sit around a lot.

● **10** Arrange to be busy over the New Year period so you don't have time to think about food. Often more weight is gained at this time because of the 'finishing up' of the Christmas leftovers. Plan a day trip or even a holiday.

CHRISTMAS SHOPPING

When purchasing goodies for the family in the run-up to Christmas, do bear in mind whether they really need them. If you still decide to go ahead, try to select low-fat foods in preference to high-fat varieties.

Here is my Traffic Light Guide to Christmas goodies:

GREEN	AMBER	RED
All vegetables cooked without fat	Vegetables cooked in fat	Roast potatoes cooked in fat
Turkey (no skin)	Goose (no skin)	Any poultry cooked or served with butter or skin
Gravy, with all fat removed	Turkey with skin	
Low-fat Christmas Pudding (see recipes, page 161)	Nuts in shells	Gravy made with fat
Low-fat Brandy Sauce (see recipe, page 164)	Regular mince pies, Christmas pudding, brandy sauce, Christmas cake without marzipan	Christmas cake with marzipan
Low-fat Mince pies – 1 only (see recipe, page 168)	Tropical Fruit Cake (see recipe, page 165)	Brandy butter
Christmas Ring (see recipe, page 164) in moderation	Festive Fruit Crunch (see recipe, page 165)	Marzipan
Ice Cream Sponge (see recipe, page 164) in moderation	Honey Fruits (see recipe, page 166)	Pies
Raisin and Orange Loaf (see recipe, page 165)	Lemon and Orange Creams (see recipe, page 166)	Quiches
Swiss Roll (see recipe, page 166)	Snowflakes (see recipe, page 166)	Pastries
Dates in moderation	Melting Mallows (see recipe, page 167)	Cream
Roast chestnuts	Mint Creams (see recipe, page 167)	Biscuits
Crystallised ginger	Raisin Rolls (see recipe, page 167)	Peanuts
Marshmallows		Shelled nuts
Orange and lemon slices		Buttered brazils
Turkish Delight		Chocolate brazils
		Chocolates
		Chocolate liqueurs
		Sugared almonds
		Fudge
		Toffees
		Caramel
		Butterscotch

CHRISTMAS DAY

ALL PORTIONS ARE ONE PER PERSON

BREAKFAST

½ a melon topped with 4 oz (100g) grapes, washed and pipped, plus 5 oz (125g) melon-flavoured diet yogurt

OR

6 oz (150g) fresh fruit salad topped with 5 oz (125g) diet yogurt, any flavour

LUNCH

Prawn Cocktail (see Christmas Day recipe, page 159)

Roast Turkey (see Christmas Day recipe, page 159)

Bread Sauce (see Christmas Day recipe, page 160)

Cranberry sauce (from jar – any brand)

Celery, Apricot and Chestnut Stuffing (see Christmas Day recipe, page 160)

Brussels Sprouts with Chestnuts (see Christmas Day recipe, page 160)

Carrots, Peas, Sweetcorn and Mange Tout (see Christmas Day recipe, page 161)

Dry-roast Potatoes (see recipe, page 134)

Gravy (see Roast Turkey recipe, page 159)

Ginger Sorbet (see recipe, page 137)

Christmas Pudding with Brandy Sauce (see Christmas Day recipes, pages 161 and 164)

OR

Ice Cream Sponge (see Christmas Day recipe, page 164)

Coffee

SUPPER

Cold turkey and ham (with all skin and fat removed)

Mixed salad served with Reduced-Oil Dressing (see recipe, page 146)

Branston pickle (1 dessertspoon per person)

Raspberry Surprise (see Christmas Day recipe, page 164)

OR

Christmas Ring (see Christmas Day recipe, page 164)

OR

Raisin and Orange Loaf (see Christmas Day recipe, page 165)

OR

Festive Fruit Crunch (see Christmas Day recipe, page 165)

CHRISTMAS DRINKS

Pre-lunch:

Grapefruit Fizz – unlimited (see Christmas Day recipe, page 166)

OR

St Clements – unlimited (see Christmas Day recipe, page 166)

Lunch:

White wine or champagne – 2 glasses per person

Spritzer – 4 glasses per person allowed (see Christmas Day recipe, page 166)

Sparkling mineral water – unlimited

Dessert:

Port – 1 small glass per person allowed

Coffee (preferably decaffeinated) with skimmed milk

CHRISTMAS DAY RECIPES

PRAWN COCKTAIL

3 oz (75g) shelled prawns per
person
lettuce
fresh lemon

Wash the prawns carefully and drain well. Wash the lettuce leaves and shred finely. Place the shredded lettuce in a stemmed wine or champagne glass to cover the bottom of the glass. Place the prawns on top and store in a cool place.

Dress with the sauce just before serving and decorate by sprinkling paprika on top and by wedging a slice of lemon on the rim of the glass.

PRAWN COCKTAIL SAUCE

(ALLOW THE
FOLLOWING AMOUNTS
PER PERSON)

1 tablespoon tomato ketchup
½ tablespoon reduced-oil,
low-calorie salad dressing
freshly ground black pepper
to taste
dash Tabasco sauce
1 tablespoon natural yogurt

Mix all the ingredients together and store in a refrigerator until needed.

ROAST TURKEY

(SERVES 8–10)

12 lbs (5.4kg) fresh turkey
Celery, Apricot and Chestnut
Stuffing (see recipe page 160)
1 pint (500ml) chicken stock
2 tablespoons gravy powder
2 chicken stock cubes or stock
made from turkey giblets

Wash the turkey thoroughly in cold water and remove the giblets and any fat. Fill the neck end with the Celery, Apricot and Chestnut Stuffing mixture. Use no fat.

Pour 1 pint (500ml) of chicken stock into a large roasting tin and place the turkey on a wire rack. Cover with tin foil and place in a preheated oven (180°C, 350°F, or Gas Mark 4), allowing a cooking time of 15 minutes per lb (0.5kg) plus 20 minutes over. (A larger bird, weighing in excess of 14 lbs (6.3kg), should be cooked for 12 minutes per lb (0.5kg) with 20 minutes over.)

Turn the roasting tin round every hour to ensure even cooking. One hour before serving, remove the turkey from the oven and place the tin foil to one side for later use. Pour off

most of the liquid from the roasting tin into a large bowl or jug. Return the turkey (without the foil) to the oven for 30 minutes.

Meanwhile, place 4 large icecubes in the turkey liquid. After 5 minutes place the liquid in the refrigerator or deep-freeze in order to cool it as fast as possible. The fat will then separate and thicken, allowing it to be removed before you make the gravy.

Mix 2 tablespoons gravy powder (not granules) with ¼ pint (125ml) cold water and add 2 chicken stock cubes or home-made turkey stock — made by boiling the turkey giblets in water for 45 minutes. This should be allowed to cool and all fat removed before use in either gravy or soup. Keep the uncooked gravy mixture to one side awaiting separated turkey liquid and strained vegetable water from cooked vegetables (see page 161).

Thirty minutes before serving, remove the turkey from the oven and pierce one of the legs with a skewer or sharp knife. If the juice that runs out is clear the bird is cooked, but if the juice is coloured with blood, return the turkey to the oven for a little longer.

When cooked, remove the turkey from the oven and place in a warm place for 30 minutes, replacing the tin foil over the bird to keep it moist and warm. This 'resting time' makes carving much easier.

To make the gravy: Add the separated turkey liquid and strained vegetable water to the uncooked gravy mixture. Bring to the boil, then simmer until ready to serve.

BREAD SAUCE

(SERVES 6–8)

½ pint (250ml) skimmed milk
1 small onion, chopped
3 cloves
1 bay leaf
6–8 tablespoons fresh breadcrumbs
freshly ground black pepper

Slowly bring the milk to the boil and add the chopped onion, cloves and bay leaf. Remove from heat, cover the pan and leave to one side for 15–20 minutes to allow the flavours to infuse.

Remove the cloves and bay leaf, add the breadcrumbs and black pepper and return to the heat. Stir gently until boiling, then remove from the heat and place in a small, covered serving dish. (A small bowl covered with tin foil would work just as well.) Keep warm until ready to serve.

CELERY, APRICOT AND CHESTNUT STUFFING

(SERVES 8–10)

1 head celery
3 oz (75g) dried apricots, soaked overnight, or 4 oz (100g) no-soak apricots
6 oz (150g) chestnuts, fresh or canned
2 medium onions
1½ wine glasses white wine
4 oz (100g) fresh breadcrumbs
1 tablespoon parsley, preferably fresh
salt and freshly ground black pepper

Prepare the ingredients by washing and trimming the celery and chopping it finely. Chop each apricot into 4 or 5 pieces. Blanch the chestnuts in boiling water for 2 minutes, and peel the skin off while hot. Peel and chop the onions.

Dry-fry the onions in a non-stick frying pan until soft and brown. Add the wine, celery, apricots and chestnuts. Cook over a brisk heat for about 4 minutes, stirring continuously. Remove from the heat and place the contents of the pan into a large bowl and allow to cool.

When cool, add the breadcrumbs, parsley, salt and pepper. The combined mixture should be firm. Add more breadcrumbs or wine if necessary.

The mixture is now ready to be used to stuff the turkey (see recipe for Roast Turkey, page 159).

BRUSSELS SPROUTS WITH CHESTNUTS

(SERVES 6–8)

1 lb (400g) chestnuts
1–2 lbs (400–800g) Brussels sprouts
¾ pint (375ml) chicken stock
freshly ground black pepper

Skin the chestnuts by blanching them quickly in boiling water for 2 minutes, then peeling off the skin while hot.

Trim and wash the sprouts and cook in boiling salted water until just tender.

Place the chestnuts in a small saucepan with the stock. Cover and cook until soft and the stock has been absorbed.

Gently mix the chestnuts with the sprouts in a serving dish and sprinkle with black pepper. Cover and keep warm until ready to serve.

CARROTS, PEAS, SWEETCORN AND MANGE TOUT

·····························

(UNLIMITED QUANTITY)

Slice the carrots into small sticks and cook until just tender, taking care not to overcook them.

Then place the peas and sweetcorn together in boiling water and simmer for only 5 minutes.

Trim and wash the mange tout. Place in boiling salted water and cook for 3 minutes.

Drain all the vegetables, mix together and place in a covered serving dish. Keep warm until ready to serve.

(Reserve all strained vegetable water for use in gravy to go with Roast Turkey [see recipe, page 159] and any Turkey Soup [see recipe, page 168] that may you make for Boxing Day.)

LIGHT CHRISTMAS PUDDING

·····························

(IDEAL FOR AN INDIVIDUAL PORTION)

Line the bottom of a dish with mincemeat (use the recipe for Spicy Fat-free Mincemeat, see Boxing Day recipe, page 168). Sprinkle a layer of fine breadcrumbs or porridge oats (approximately 2 oz [50g]) on top and then sprinkle 1 tablespoon of sugar over.

Microwave on high for 2 minutes and then place under a hot grill until the breadcrumbs are brown and crispy.

Serve immediately.

CHRISTMAS PUDDING

·····························

(SERVES 8–10)

3 oz (75g) currants
3 oz (75g) sultanas
4 oz (100g) raisins
4 tablespoons brandy, rum or beer
3 oz (75g) glacé cherries, halved
3 oz (75g) plain or self-raising flour
1 teaspoon mixed spice
½ teaspoon cinnamon
2 oz (50g) fresh breadcrumbs
2 oz (50g) muscovado or caster sugar
2 teaspoons gravy browning
rind of ½ lemon and ½ orange, grated
4 oz (100g) apple, grated
4 oz (100g) carrot, finely grated
1 tablespoon lemon juice
2 eggs
4 tablespoons milk
2 tablespoons molasses or cane sugar syrup
extra rum or brandy

Soak the dried fruit in the rum, brandy or beer, and leave overnight.

When ready to make the pudding, shake the halved cherries in the flour, then add all the other dry ingredients, plus the gravy browning. Mix in the peel (rind), grated apple and carrot, and lemon juice. Beat the eggs with the milk and molasses or cane sugar syrup and slowly add to the mixture. Mix together gently and thoroughly.

Place in a 2-pint (1 litre) ovenproof basin and cook by microwaving or steaming, as follows. Microwave on high (with an upturned plate over the basin) for 5 minutes, leave to rest for 5 minutes, then microwave for another 5 minutes. Alternatively, steam gently for 3 hours. This makes a more moist pudding.

After cooking, allow the pudding to cool, then wrap in tin foil until required. Before reheating, pierce pudding with a fork and add 4 additional tablespoons of rum or brandy. Steam for 1–2 hours.

This pudding can be deep-frozen. Thaw thoroughly before reheating.

Overleaf: Roast Turkey; Bread Sauce; Brussels Sprouts with Chestnuts; Carrots, Peas, Sweetcorn and Mange-Tout

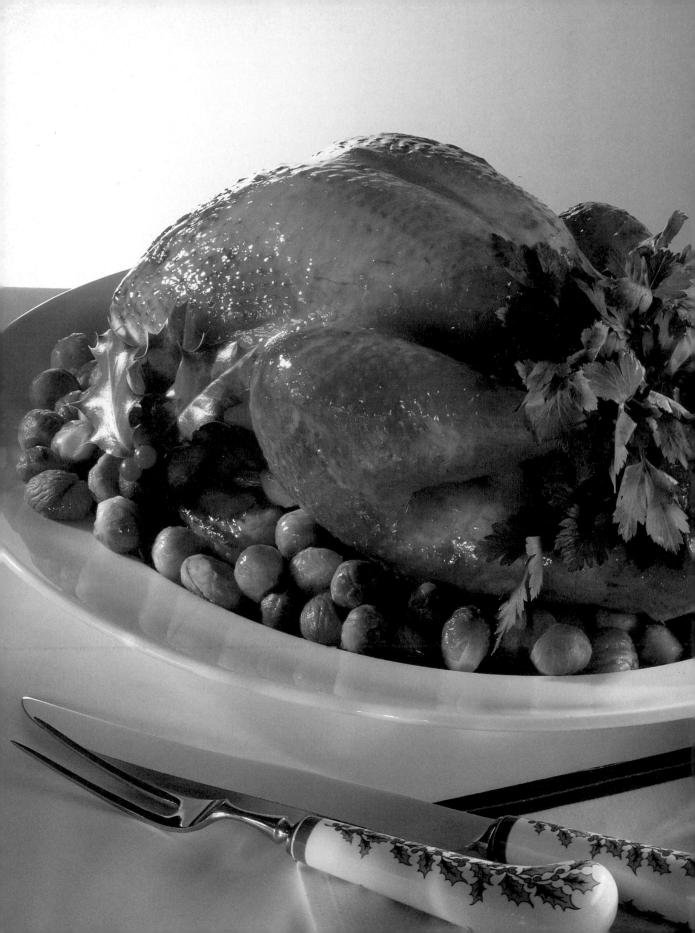

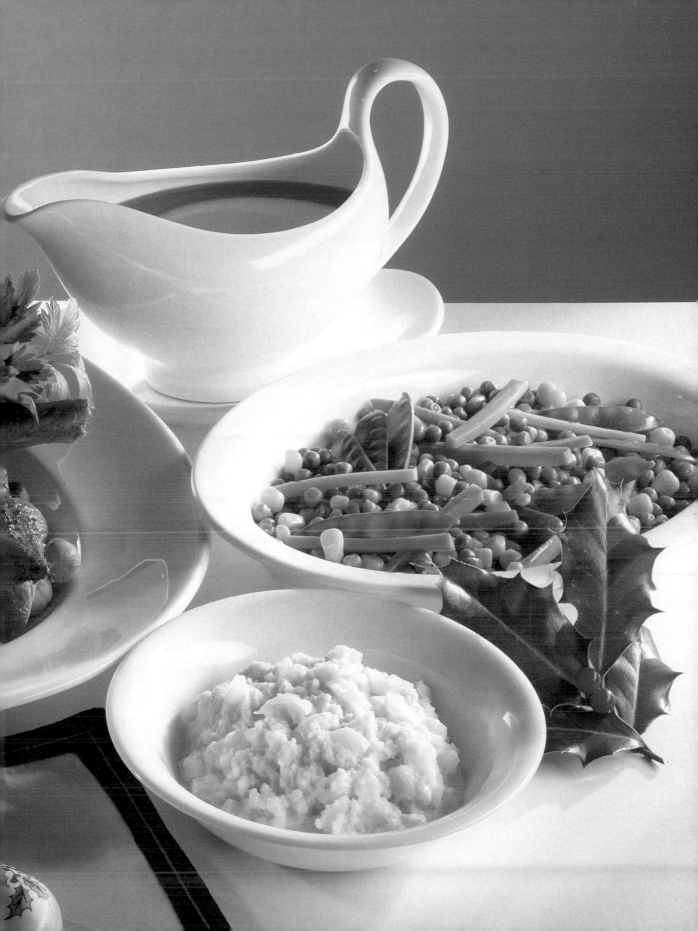

BRANDY SAUCE

....

1 pint (500ml) skimmed milk
3 drops almond essence
2 tablespoons cornflour
liquid artificial sweetener
3 tablespoons brandy

Heat all but 4 tablespoons of the milk with the almond essence until almost boiling and remove from the heat. Mix the cornflour and remaining cold milk thoroughly and slowly pour it into the hot milk, stirring continuously until the mixture begins to thicken. Return to the heat and bring to the boil. Continue to cook, stirring all the time. If it is too thin, mix some more cornflour with cold milk and add it slowly until you achieve the consistency of custard. Sweeten to taste. Add the brandy a few drops at a time and stir well. Cover the serving jug and keep warm until ready to serve.

RASPBERRY SURPRISE

....

(SERVES 6)

16 oz (400g) frozen
raspberries
4 × 5 oz (4 × 125g)
raspberry-flavoured yogurts

Thaw the raspberries slowly in a refrigerator and reserve 6 well-shaped raspberries for decoration. Place yogurt in a large bowl and gently stir in the raspberries.

Spoon the mixture into stemmed wineglasses and place a raspberry on the top of each. Store in the refrigerator until ready to serve.

ICE CREAM SPONGE

....

(SERVES 6)

For the sponge
2 eggs
3 oz (75g) caster sugar
3 oz (75g) self-raising flour, sifted
For the filling
1 family brick low-fat vanilla ice cream
1 lb (400g) any tinned fruit in natural juice, or sufficient fresh or frozen fruit to generously fill the sponge

To make this fat-free sponge, first whisk together the eggs and sugar for several minutes until you have a thick, pale consistency. Then carefully fold in the sifted flour.

Place in a 7-inch (17.5cm) cake tin lined with parchment paper and bake in a moderate oven (180°C, 350°F, or Gas Mark 4) for 30 minutes, or until golden brown. Leave in the cake tin for 5 minutes, then turn out on to a wire rack and allow to cool completely.

To serve, slice the cake into 3 horizontal layers and spread each layer with ice cream and fruit before reassembling.

CHRISTMAS RING

....

(SERVES 6–8)

This is a low-fat scone mixture with a fruity filling that can be formed into a ring and decorated to make a festive treat.

For scone mixture
1½ oz (37.5g) very low-fat spread
8 oz (200g) self-raising flour
2 oz (50g) soft brown sugar
1 egg
5 tablespoons skimmed milk
For the filling
1 oz (25g) sugar
6 oz (150g) mixed dried fruit
1 teaspoon mixed spice
1 tablespoon lemon juice or brandy
For decoration
8 oz (200g) icing sugar
orange juice to mix

Using your fingers, rub in the very low-fat spread with the flour in a large bowl. Add the sugar and mix well. In a separate small bowl beat the egg and milk together, then mix into the content of the large bowl to form a dough. Roll out into a rectangle, approximately 7 × 14 inches (17 × 35 cm).

To make the filling, stir the sugar, dried fruit and mixed spice together and spread evenly over the scone mixture. Sprinkle liberally with lemon juice or brandy.

Using your fingers, roll up the 14-inch (35cm) side of the dough to form a long thin sausage shape, and then bring the two ends together to form a ring shape. Place on to a baking tray lined with parchment paper. Bake at 200°C, 400°F, or Gas Mark 7 for 20-25 minutes. Leave to cool.

To serve, arrange shapes of holly, Christmas bells, stars or bows (all made out of icing) on the ring to give it a garland effect. Alternatively, mix icing sugar with orange juice and glaze the top of the ring.

RAISIN AND ORANGE LOAF

....

(1 SERVING = ½ INCH [1.25CM] SLICE)

8 oz (200g) self-raising flour
6 oz (150g) raisins
4 oz (100g) soft brown sugar
1 egg, beaten
grated rind and juice of orange made up with milk to ½ pint (250ml) liquid

Mix all the ingredients together well and place in a lined 2-lb (800g) loaf tin. Bake in a cool oven (170°C, 320°F, or Gas Mark 3) for 1½ hours or until cooked.

FESTIVE FRUIT CRUNCH

....

(MAKES 15–20 SQUARES)

8 oz (200g) mincemeat (preferably without fat, or use Spicy Fat-free Mincemeat, see Boxing Day recipe, page 168)
4 oz (100g) cornflakes
9 oz (225g) dried fruit
2 eggs
1 level teaspoon mixed spice
14 oz (350g) tin Fussel's condensed milk (made with skimmed milk)
2 oz (50g) chopped walnuts or 2 oz (50g) glacé cherries, quartered

Mix all the ingredients together and place in a 7–8inch (17.5–20cm) lined square cake tin. Bake in the oven at 150°C, 300°F, or Gas Mark 2 for approximately 1¼ hours until firm to the touch. Leave in the tin to cool, then cut into squares or chunks to serve.

TROPICAL FRUIT CAKE

....

(1 SERVING = ½ INCH [1.25CM] SLICE)

3 ripe bananas
2 large carrots
2 eggs
6 oz (150g) soft brown sugar
8 oz (200g) self-raising flour
1 teaspoon mixed spice
1 teaspoon vanilla essence
5 oz (125g) tinned apricots, in natural juice, drained (reserve juice for topping)

Mash the bananas, and peel and grate the carrots. Mix together all the ingredients and place in a lined 2-lb (1kg) cake tin. Bake in a preheated oven at 190°C, 375°F, Gas Mark 5 for approximately 50 minutes.

When cool, either spread the top with apricot fromage frais (if the cake is going to be eaten the same day) or with icing made by mixing icing sugar with the juice from the tinned apricots.

SWISS ROLL

(SERVES 8)

Use the same sponge mixture as for 'Ice Cream Sponge' (see Christmas Day recipe, page 164) but bake in a Swiss roll tin at 220°C, 425°F, or Gas Mark 7 for 7 minutes.

Turn out while still warm on to sugared greaseproof paper. Spread with jam and roll up the long side using fingers and the paper. Leave to cool with paper wrapped around the roll.

For extra-special occasions, spread with fromage frais and soft fresh fruit.

DRINKS

GRAPEFRUIT FIZZ

unsweetened grapefruit juice
slimline tonic water

Pour approximately 4 fl oz (100ml) unsweetened grapefruit juice into a tall glass and add plenty of ice. Add slimline tonic to taste, and top up with the remainder of the tonic when required.

ST CLEMENTS

slimline orange
slimline bitter lemon

Pour half a bottle of each into a tall glass filled with ice. Top up as required.

To make it even more delicious, use freshly squeezed orange juice with the bitter lemon.

SPRITZER

2½ fl oz (62.5ml) white wine
sparkling mineral water or
soda water

Pour the wine into a wineglass and add the mineral or soda water.

SWEETS

SNOWFLAKES

1 egg white
3 oz icing sugar

Put the egg white in a bowl and stir the icing sugar into it. Place the bowl over a saucepan of boiling water and whisk the mixture until it is thick and stands up in peaks. Remove from the heat and beat for a

further minute. Place in spoonfuls on to parchment paper and flatten slightly. Leave to set for 24 hours in a cool place.

HONEY FRUITS

3 oz (75g) stoned dates
3 oz (75g) walnuts
4 oz (100g) dried mixed fruit
2 teaspoons honey
icing sugar

Chop the dates and walnuts and mix together. Add the dried fruit and honey, mix well and make into little balls. Roll them in icing sugar until well covered.

NB Although nuts are not usually allowed, I have included this recipe as a special Christmas treat.

LEMON AND ORANGE CREAMS

1 small orange
8 oz (200g) icing sugar
orange or lemon candied slices

Grate the rind of the orange and squeeze the juice. Add about 4 teaspoons of juice and all the rind to the icing sugar and mix well. Place on to a board, roll out and cut into shapes. Place an orange or lemon slice on top of each.

MELTING MALLOWS

....

2 oz (50g) marshmallows
4 oz (100g) icing sugar
2 oz (50g) glacé cherries or mixed glacé fruits, chopped
extra icing sugar

Melt marshmallows in a bowl over a saucepan of boiling water, add the icing sugar and the cherries and mix well. Knead into a large roll on a surface dusted with the extra icing sugar. Roll out and cut into ½-inch (1.25cm) squares.

MINT CREAMS

....

8 oz (200g) icing sugar
few drops peppermint essence
4 teaspoons hot water
green food colouring
extra icing sugar

Mix the icing sugar with the peppermint essence and hot water. Divide in half and add 1 or 2 drops of green food colouring to one half only. Knead both halves separately on a board dusted with the extra icing sugar. Roll out and cut into shapes. Alternatively, mix the green half with the white half before rolling out, to give a marbled effect.

RAISIN ROLLS

....

4 oz (100g) marshmallows
1 oz (25g) raisins chopped
1½ oz (37.5g) Rice Krispies

Melt the marshmallows in a bowl placed over a pan of boiling water. Remove from the heat and add the raisins and Rice Krispies. Make into little balls using your hands or a spoon and place on a baking tray lined with parchment.

If you find that the mixture is very sticky, wet your hands or the spoon before shaping it into balls.

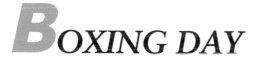

BOXING DAY

....

(ALL PORTIONS ARE PER PERSON)

BREAKFAST

- 6 oz (150g) fresh fruit salad topped with 5 oz (125g) diet yogurt, any flavour

LUNCH

- Turkey Soup (see Boxing Day recipe, page 168)
- Jacket potato served with salad and 4 oz (100g) of cooked turkey plus 1 tablespoon Branston pickle

TEA

- 2 slices wholemeal bread spread with low-fat salad dressing and made into open sandwiches with chopped salad, topped with 1 oz (25g) ham, cut into strips, or 2 oz (50g) prawns
- 2 low-fat mince pies – use the recipe for Spicy Fat-free Mincemeat (see Boxing Day recipe, page 168)

OR

- Pineapple and Orange Sorbet (see Boxing Day recipe, page 168) and 1 low-fat mince pie

BOXING DAY RECIPES

TURKEY SOUP

(SERVES 4)

bones of one turkey
vegetable water (enough to
cover the bones)
any remaining gravy
bouquet garni
freshly ground black pepper
2 chicken stock cubes
10 black peppercorns
2 bay leaves

Remove all skin from the turkey bones and place them in a very large saucepan. Break the turkey carcass in the middle to help it to fit into the saucepan if necessary. Pour the vegetable water over the bones and add all other ingredients.

Bring to the boil, cover and simmer for 2–3 hours. Taste and add additional seasoning if required. If the flavour is too weak, continue cooking for longer. Strain and, when cool, place in the refrigerator so that any fat comes to the top. When the fat solidifies, remove it, and the turkey soup is then ready for reheating when required.

SPICY FAT-FREE MINCEMEAT

(MAKES 3¾lbs [1.7kg])

2 lbs (800g) mixed fruit
1¼ lbs (500g) cooking apples,
peeled and grated
2 teaspoons mixed spice
1 pint (500ml) sweet cider
2 tablespoons brandy, whisky
or rum

The occasional mince pie at Christmas time is a treat we can all enjoy. To make it as low in fat as possible, use the above ingredients for fat-free mincemeat.

Put the dried fruit in a saucepan with the grated apple, spice and cider. Simmer for about 20 minutes or until it has formed a pulp and most of the liquid has evaporated. Stir in your choice of spirit.

Pack into sterilised jars and store in a fridge until required. It will keep in a fridge for 4 months. Once opened, use within one week.

PINEAPPLE AND ORANGE SORBET

(SERVES 6)

small tin crushed pineapple in
natural juice
1 orange, peeled and chopped
8 fl oz (200ml) fresh orange
juice
liquid artificial sweetener
2 egg whites

Crush pineapple well and mix with chopped orange and orange juice. Sweeten to taste. Place in a plastic container in your freezer or the freezer compartment of your refrigerator. Freeze until half-frozen.

Whisk egg whites until stiff. Turn out half-frozen mixture into a bowl, mash it to an even consistency, then fold in the egg whites.

Return mixture to freezer until firm.

NEW YEAR'S EVE PARTY

- Garlic Bread (8 × quantity given in recipe, see below)
- Cold Prawn and Rice Salad (see recipe, page 120)
- Tuna Pâté with Crudités (see recipe, page 99)
- Ham, Beef and Chicken or Turkey Salad (see recipe, page 104)
- Scone Vol-au-Vents with various fillings (see New Year recipe, page 170)
- 2 lettuces
- 2 cucumbers
- 2 endives
- 1 lb (400g) grated carrots mixed with 4 oz (100g) sultanas
- 3 lbs (1.2kg) tomatoes
- 1 head celery
- Reduced-Oil Dressing (see recipe, page 146)
- fresh fruit salad (3 oranges, 3 apples, 3 pears, 2 kiwifruits, 4 oz [100g] black grapes, 4 oz [100g] green grapes, ½ pineapple, 2 bananas, mixed with 5 fl oz [125g] unsweetened orange juice).
- Mango and Strawberry Bombe (double quantity of recipe, see page 138), served with different flavours of diet yogurt or fromage frais
- Fresh Pineapple in Kirsch (double quantity of recipe, see page 170), served with different flavours of diet yogurt or fromage frais.

DRINKS

- white wine
- champagne (allow half a bottle per person)

And for those who don't want to drink and drive:
- slimline drinks
- sparkling apple or grape juice
- sparkling mineral water
- Pacific Delight (see recipe, page 170)
- Sludge Gulper (see recipe, page 170)

General guidelines: serve the Garlic Bread half an hour before the main buffet. Everything can be prepared well in advance and the host(s) can relax and enjoy the evening, knowing that the food can be served when everyone is ready to eat.

NEW YEAR'S EVE PARTY RECIPES

GARLIC BREAD

4 oz (100g) very low-fat spread
4 cloves fresh garlic, crushed
1 teaspoon lemon juice
1 French loaf
salt

Mix the very low-fat spread with the garlic and lemon juice. Cut the loaf into ¾ inch (1.8cm) slices, slanting the knife diagonally across the loaf. Spread each slice with the garlic mixture, re-form the loaf and sprinkle salt across the top. Wrap in tin foil and place in a preheated hot oven at 220°C, 425°F, or Gas Mark 7 for 10 minutes. Serve immediately.

SCONE VOL-AU-VENTS

....

*(MAKES
APPROXIMATELY 12
VOL-AU-VENTS)*

For scone mixture
*1½ oz (37.5g) very low-fat
spread*
8 oz (200g) self-raising flour
1 teaspoon mixed herbs
8 tablespoons milk

Fillings
Cottage cheese mixed with prawns and Marie-Rose dressing (see recipe, page 146) *or* ham pieces mixed with low-fat soft cheese spread *or* tuna, cucumber and natural yogurt or reduced-oil salad dressing *or* cold chicken, diced and mixed with yogurt or reduced-oil salad dressing and a touch of curry paste.

Using your fingers, rub the very low-fat spread into the flour and stir in the mixed herbs. Add the milk and mix well to form a dough. Roll out, then, using a 2-inch (5cm) round cutter, cut out rounds. Then cut gently into the centre of each round using a smaller cutter (1 inch/2.5cm), without cutting right through the dough. This forms the hollows in the vol-au-vents.

Place on a baking sheet and bake in a hot oven (220°C, 425°F, or Gas Mark 7) for 12–15 minutes. Allow to cool, then scoop out the vol-au-vent centres.

To serve, fill generously with any of the fillings suggested above.

FRESH PINEAPPLE IN KIRSCH

....

(SERVES 4)

1 large fresh pineapple
*1 liqueur/sherry glass of
Kirsch*

Remove the skin from the pineapple and slice the flesh into rings. Remove the central core from each slice with a small pastry cutter. Place the pineapple rings in a glass serving dish. Pour the Kirsch over and place in a refrigerator for 6 hours to marinate. Turn the fruit occasionally to ensure even flavouring.

Serve chilled.

TROPICAL FRUIT SALAD

....

(SERVES 4)

6 oz (150g) fresh pineapple
1 mango
1 banana
1 kiwifruit
2 oranges

4 oz (100g) seedless grapes
*6 fl oz (150ml) tropical fruit
juice*
*2 fl oz (50ml) fruit liqueur,
e.g. Grand Marnier,
Cointreau or Kirsch (optional)*

Using a sharp knife, remove the skin from the pineapple. Cut into half and remove the hard core. Cut out the flesh and cut into cubes. Peel and slice the mango, banana and kiwifruit into small bite-sized pieces. Peel the oranges and remove all the pith, then chop into small pieces.

Mix all the ingredients together, place in the refrigerator and serve within 1 hour to avoid discoloration.

DRINKS

PACIFIC DELIGHT

....

Mix 2 fl oz (50ml) lime cordial with slimline ginger ale in a tall glass filled with ice.

SLUDGE GULPER

....

Pour 4 fl oz (100ml) unsweetened orange juice into a tall glass filled with ice. Add the diet coke.

CHRISTMAS BINGE CORRECTOR DIET

Christmas is undoubtedly the time when most people gain weight and whilst I have named this the Christmas Binge Corrector Diet accordingly, it is also suitable for counteracting the results of any other period of over-indulgence. Whatever the cause, it is essential that, firstly, you go on this corrector diet immediately after your over-indulgence (leaving it a week will not have the same effect), and, secondly, that you do not follow it for more than the recommended two days. If you *do*, you will bring your metabolic rate down and will regain your lost weight when you stop. Two days is, I believe, the *maximum* period we can go on a lower-calorie diet without adversely affecting our metabolism. By following this short, sharp, two-day plan you will be amazed how much of your gained weight disappears.

DAY 1

DAILY ALLOWANCE:

8 fl oz (250ml) skimmed or semi-skimmed milk

BREAKFAST

- 1 whole fresh grapefruit
- glass of sparkling mineral water

LUNCH

- Large salad of lettuce, cucumber, tomatoes, grated carrot, grated cabbage, watercress, plus 1 oz (25g) cooked chicken/ham/turkey or 2 oz (50g) cottage cheese, with oil-free Citrus Dressing (see recipe, page 146)
- 5 oz (125g) diet yogurt

DINNER

- 4 oz (100g) white fish or 2 oz (50g) cooked chicken, served with 12 oz (300g) vegetables (e.g. carrots, cabbage, cauliflower, spinach, broccoli, celery), plus 2 tablespoons tomato sauce (for the fish) or 3 fl oz (75ml) thin gravy (with the chicken)
- 1 piece fresh fruit

DAY 2

DAILY ALLOWANCE:

10 fl oz (250ml) skimmed or semi-skimmed milk

BREAKFAST

- 1 Weetabix or 1 oz (25g) Allbran, 1 teaspoon sugar, and milk from allowance
- glass of sparkling mineral water

LUNCH

- 5 fl oz (125ml) unsweetened fruit juice
- 1 slimmer's cup-a-soup plus 1 slice light wholemeal bread (e.g. Nimble or Slimcea)
- 5 oz (125g) diet yogurt plus 1 piece fresh fruit

DINNER

- 3 oz (75g) chicken (no skin), served with unlimited vegetables (e.g. carrots, cabbage, cauliflower, spinach, broccoli, celery) plus a little thin gravy
- 1 piece any fresh fruit

A HEALTHIER, HAPPIER PREGNANCY

Having a baby is often the cause of many women becoming overweight for the first time in their lives. This is a great shame because it need not be so. There is no doubt that during pregnancy the body undergoes some dramatic changes – both metabolic and structural. For instance, a meal that would normally satisfy our appetite for 4–5 hours can be burned up in just two, leaving us ravenous. Physically, too, our body becomes more flexible. This is due to our ligaments increasing in elasticity and some of the joints becoming more mobile to allow for the growing foetus and the forthcoming birth itself. In the later stages of pregnancy the main abdominal muscle (rectus abdominis) can actually split and separate to accommodate our 'bulge'. In most cases it will come together again after the baby is born, and a flat abdomen can be achieved once more.

Keeping weight gain to a minimum during pregnancy will help to prevent problems we can well do without once the baby is born. After the birth our body has quite enough readjusting to do as well as coping with the increased physical demands of caring for a new-born baby, without having to cope with the extra burden of carrying around several stones or kilograms of excess weight. It is totally natural to feel tired, if not exhausted, in the weeks after giving birth, but the prospect of having to *continue* to wear maternity clothes because none of the others in your wardrobe fit you can be particularly depressing. It is inadvisable to diet too soon after having your baby, especially if breastfeeding, so it is infinitely preferable not to gain an excessive amount of weight during pregnancy. The medical profession recommends that no more than 20–28 lbs (9–12.7kg) should be gained. As soon as the baby is born we lose about 14 lbs (6.4kg) – this varies according to the size of the baby, of course and the rest of the weight is usually some fluid, which goes in approximately one week, and fat.

Breastfeeding not only supplies your baby with lots of valuable nutritious calories as well as antibodies, it also causes you to burn lots of calories in producing and supplying the milk. Breastfeeding also helps the uterus (womb) to return to normal more quickly, and may help you to regain your figure earlier. Unfortunately, for a variety of reasons not all women are able to breastfeed their babies. They may not be physically able to produce adequate milk; the breasts may not be functioning satisfactorily, or the baby might find taking milk from the breast difficult. Also, mothers who have to leave their babies while they go to work may find a bottle is a more convenient alternative. Mothers who bottle-feed their babies may find it harder to regain their figures than those who breastfeed. However, it *can* still be achieved.

Your doctor and midwife will give you all the advice and help you need to keep you healthy throughout pregnancy, and afterwards. However, here are a few guidelines on sensible eating that will keep your weight gain at a reasonable level so that you are less likely to have an overweight problem after your baby is born.

If you are overweight *before* you become pregnant, weight gain during pregnancy should be kept to a minimum. Before I became pregnant with my daughter Dawn, I weighed 9 stones (57kg), which was a stone (6.3kg) overweight for me. I gained only 12 lbs (5.4kg) throughout my pregnancy, and a few weeks after Dawn was born I weighed only 8 st 3 lbs (52.2kg). Not only did I feel much fitter at this lighter weight, I also felt so much better and happier. I breastfed her for a year and avoided postnatal depression. For me, having a baby was the most wonderful experience of my life. I ate only healthy nutritious foods throughout my pregnancy and avoided all high-fat and junk foods. In my case, I believe this was the key to preventing an overweight problem.

Here is my Traffic Light Guide to eating healthily during pregnancy.

AMBER

The following foods should be consumed in moderation:
- Very low-fat spreads
- Jams, marmalades, honey
- Full-cream milk
- Custards and milk puddings
- Ice cream (not Cornish varieties)
- Gouda and Edam cheeses low-fat hard cheeses
- Vegetable oils (only very small quantities)
- Low-fat mayonnaise
- Low-fat sausages
- Dried fruit
- Low-fat cakes
- Sugar
- Alcohol (no more than 1 unit per day)

GREEN

The following foods are recommended to be eaten freely during pregnancy:
- All lean meat
- Fish
- Poultry
- Eggs
- Vegetables
- Fruit
- Semi-skimmed milk
- Cottage cheese, Quark
- Yogurts, fromage frais
- Cereals
- Rice, pasta
- Bread
- Sauces
- Low-fat dressings

RED

Avoid the following foods:
- Any foods cooked in fat
- Butter and full-fat margarine
- Fat, lard, dripping
- Cream
- Mayonnaise
- Fatty meat products such as German sausage, pork pie, salami, sausage rolls, Scotch eggs, etc.
- Cakes and pastries
- Chocolate, sweets, fudge, toffee, etc.

NB An alternative eating plan would be to follow the guidelines in the Maintenance chapter (see page 147). However, during pregnancy avoid soft, unpasteurised cheeses, uncooked meats and some pâtés, and liver should be eaten only in small quantities.

TEN TIPS FOR A HEALTHIER PREGNANCY

- 1 As soon as you know you are pregnant make sure you start eating healthily. Follow a lower fat, but not a 'no-fat', diet. Remember, it is easier to prevent weight gain than to cure it.
- 2 Weigh and measure yourself regularly to monitor your weight and inch (centimetre) gain. Do not allow yourself to gain too much weight in the early stages of pregnancy.
- 3 Eat 3 good meals a day and try to avoid nibbling between meals.
- 4 Remove temptation from the kitchen by not re-stocking the larder with instant, high-calorie foods such as biscuits and cakes.
- 5 Always keep a supply of fresh fruit readily available. Eat this between meals only if you feel really hungry. It is preferable to keep it for mealtimes.
- 6 Stop smoking completely.
- 7 Restrict alcohol intake to a maximum of 1 unit per day (e.g. 1 small glass of wine).
- 8 Keep physically active and exercise if possible. Ask your doctor for advice here and use the BBC Pregnancy and Postnatal Exercise video.
- 9 Don't wear tight clothing or heels that are uncomfortably high. Wear a well-fitting bra to support your increased breast size.
- 10 Attend antenatal, relaxation and any pregnancy education classes. It's good to know what's happening to your body and to meet others in the same situation.

EXERCISE DURING AND AFTER PREGNANCY

Pregnancy is a physically demanding experience, and staying reasonably fit can certainly help as the day of the birth approaches. Whilst a super-fit woman is not necessarily more likely to have an easy childbirth than a woman who is unfit, being physically fit *will* help you to cope with the continuing demands of running a home.

The exercises included here are available on video (the BBC Pregnancy and Postnatal Exercise video) and have been carefully selected by obstetric physiotherapists Jane Ashton and Marjorie Polden. Jane Ashton was 8½ months into her pregnancy when we photographed her for the antenatal exercises. In addition to exercises that increase stamina, it is helpful to spend some time stretching our ligaments and muscles in preparation for the actual birth, and to strengthen muscles under stress in pregnancy.

ANTENATAL EXERCISES

Always check with your doctor or midwife *before* doing these or any other exercises.

The most important exercise for all women to do while they are pregnant and to continue after the birth of their baby is the pelvic floor exercise.

Your pelvic floor muscles are vital in supporting all your pelvic organs. They also play a part in controlling your bladder and bowels. Our pelvis is a ring or basin of bones held together by ligaments. Our pelvic floor muscles form the basin.

Although you cannot see these muscles it is just as easy to exercise them (and every bit as important) as it is to exercise the rest of your body.

The pelvic floor muscles work together as a group. This is how to recognise that you are using them: close your back passage as if you are stopping wind, close your front passage as if you are stopping the flow of urine and pull your vagina in and up as if you are gripping a tampon or plug of cotton wool. Hold this muscle contraction for as long as you can and then let your pelvic floor relax. Repeat as often as is comfortable. If your muscles are weak you may only be able to hold the contraction for as little as 3 or 4 seconds at first. With practice you should be able to increase this so that you can hold for 10 seconds or more. Aim to have 4 to 5 seconds rest between each pelvic floor squeeze. To make sure that you are working the right muscles, don't pull your but-tocks together, or your abdominal muscles in, as you exercise your pelvic floor. Even on days when you have no time for an exercise workout, try to do your pelvic floor exercises several times so that these muscles will become stronger.

Another important exercise to do during pregnancy is the pelvic tilt exercise. This strengthens your abdominal muscles and loosens your spine. You can do this while you are standing, sitting, kneeling, or lying down on your back. Curl or tilt your pelvis forwards and upwards. This will have the effect of levelling your lower back (pressing it down into the floor if you are lying on your back) and curling your pubic bone upwards. If you feel dizzy lying on your back, roll on to your side. Perform this contraction, hold for the count of 3, then slowly relax. Repeat as many times as is comfortable and at various times throughout the day.

WARMING UP

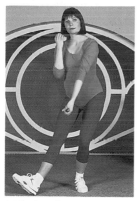 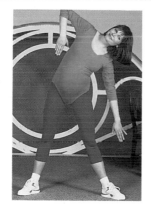 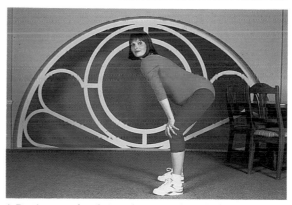

1 Flexing alternate arms, touch the floor with alternate heels. Repeat as many times as you can comfortably.

2 With feet apart and knees slightly bent, gently bend sideways extending one arm down as you bend. Curve the spine over to the side as you bend but do not twist it. Slowly straighten up and repeat to the other side. Continue repetitions to alternate sides.

Always practise the above 2 warm-up exercises before proceeding.

1 Resting your hands just above your bent knees, curve your spine downwards, pushing your seat upwards and outwards. Hold for 3 counts then curve your spine the opposite way, tilting your pelvis forwards as you do so. Hold for 3 seconds. Repeat the whole sequence 5 times in total.

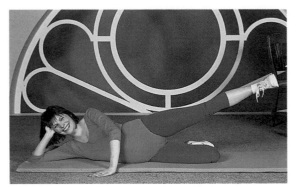

2 Lying on your side with your lower leg bent, prop your head up on your hand. Slowly raise your upper leg up and down a few inches ensuring the foot is parallel to the floor and that the leg is kept straight. Repeat as many times as is comfortable. Proceed to Exercise 3.

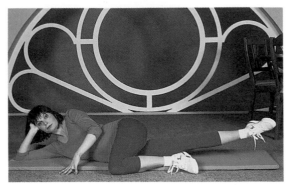

3 Lying on your side, propping your head on your hand, bend your top leg and allow it to rest on the floor in front of the lower leg. Raise the lower leg, with your knee facing forwards, as high as you can without discomfort and lower it again. Repeat the raising and lowering movement for as many times as you can in comfort.

Roll over on to your other side and repeat Exercises 2 and 3 with your other leg.

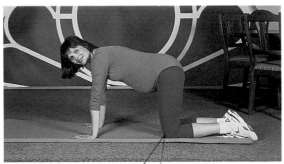

4 Position yourself on your hands and knees and practise your pelvic tilt exercises. Curl your pelvis inwards and hold for the count of 5, then relax. Repeat 5 times.

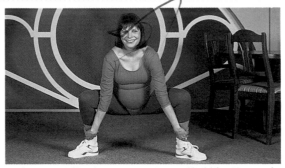

5 Place yourself in the squat position and hold for 10 seconds. Slowly stand up. Repeat the exercise once more.

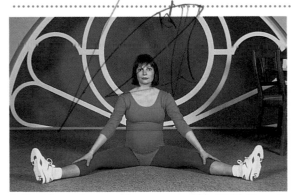

6 Sit with your legs as wide apart as possible. Hold this position for as long as you can without straining.

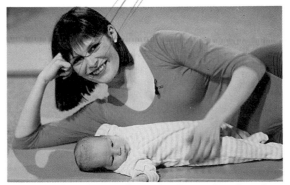

7 Relax by lying down with your head on a pillow for as long as you wish.

Jane Ashton's beautiful baby daughter arrived 9 days late weighing in at 7lbs 12 oz (3.6kg).

POSTNATAL EXERCISES

After having had their baby, many women are surprised and disappointed by their body's shape. I know I was amazed. In fact, in the maternity ward it can be quite difficult to see who has already *had* their baby! Even after the birth of the baby the abdomen will still be very distended. However, in a few days your shape will improve as things slowly get back to normal. Many physical changes take place during pregnancy and these take time to disappear. Labour and delivery of the baby will have produced further changes.

Your abdominal muscles will have been stretched and lengthened, and the two sides of your abdominal 'corset' may have split apart down the middle. The gap between the two is called the 'diastasis recti abdominis' and its width can vary from person to person.

To check how wide the gap is, lie on your back with your knees bent. Place your three middle fingers on your abdomen about one inch (2.5cm) below your waist. Now raise your head and shoulders as though you are about to sit up. You should be able to feel your two recti muscles coming together. If you have a very wide gap you will need to spread your fingers out sideways to locate and feel these muscles. The wider the gap, the

0–2 WEEKS

This series of exercises can be done with your baby. For Exercises 1 and 2 place your baby by your side on the bed and for Exercise 3, hold your baby in your arms.

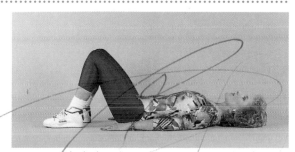

1 Lying on the bed, with your hands by your side, tilt your pelvis forwards and hold for the count of 4. As you do so, tighten the muscles in your seat. Relax and repeat 4 times. Increase the number of repetitions each day.

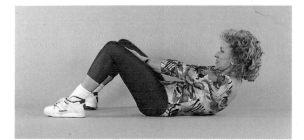

2 Lying in the same position as for Exercise 1, bend your knees. Slowly raise your head and shoulders off the bed, reaching slightly forwards with your hands towards the knees. Slowly lie down again then repeat 4 times. Increase the number of repetitions each day as you become stronger.

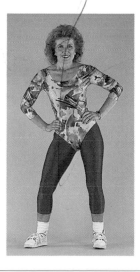

3 Sit up slowly and, after a few moments, stand up. Holding your baby in your arms if you wish, pull in your tummy and rotate your hips in an exaggerated circle. Rotate 3 times in a clockwise direction and then 3 times in an anti-clockwise direction. Increase the number of repetitions each day according to your fitness.

weaker your muscles are and the more careful you must be about introducing strong exercises. If the gap is more than two fingers in width do not practise any twisting or side-bending movements. In particular, do not practise Exercise 1 in the 2–6 Weeks section, or Exercises 2 and 4 in the 6 Weeks–4 Months section following. For alternative exercises I suggest you see the BBC Pregnancy and Postnatal video where fuller descriptions and demonstrations are given.

Before doing these or any other exercises check with your doctor or midwife.

2–6 WEEKS

Begin your exercise session with the previous exercises given for the 0–2 week period then add the following exercises to your daily workout. Hold your baby or place the baby close by you for these exercises.

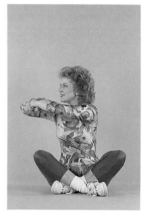

1* Sitting cross-legged with your baby in your lap, fold your arms in front of you and slowly twist from side to side, pausing in the centre before twisting to the opposite side. Repeat twice to each side. Increase the number of repetitions as you feel stronger.

*NB Avoid this exercise if your diastasis recti abdominis gap is more than two fingers in width. See the introduction to Postnatal Exercises, page 177.

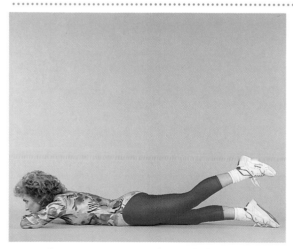

2 Lying face downwards on the floor or bed, fold your arms and place your head on your hands. Slowly raise one leg, keeping it straight. Hold for 2 counts and slowly lower it again. Repeat with the other leg. Repeat 5 times with each leg, increasing the number of repetitions as you become stronger.

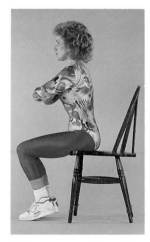

3 Sit on an upright chair, holding your baby in your arms if you wish. Sit towards the edge of the chair and sit up straight.

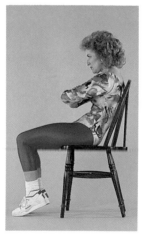

Slowly lean back in the chair, tilting your pelvis forwards as you lower your spine back into the chair. Hold for a count of 3 then slowly sit up straight again. Repeat 5 times, increasing the number of repetitions as you become stronger.

6 WEEKS – 4 MONTHS

As you become fitter and your doctor gives you permission to exercise more, the intensity of the exercises can be increased. Before a physical workout it is always important to warm up properly. Play some lively music to set a good beat and to add to your general enjoyment. If you have any other young children with you they will almost certainly enjoy working out with you.

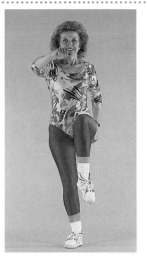

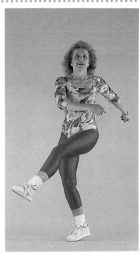

Warm-up Exercises
1 March on the spot, swinging your arms, 20 times.

2 Step then kick forwards and across with each leg in turn, 20 times, swinging your arms as you go.

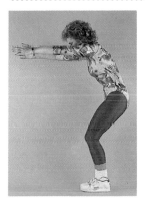

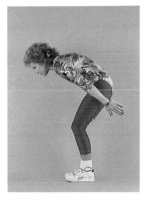

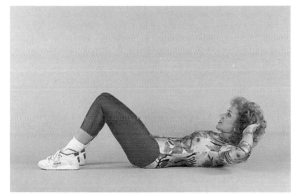

3 'Ski' down, 10 times.

Repeat these 3 warm-up exercises, in the sequence above, twice more, then proceed to the following exercises.

1 Lying on your back on the floor with your knees bent, place your hands to the sides of your head (not at the back). Raise your head, shoulders and arms a few inches towards your bent knees. Raise to the count of 3 and then return to the floor to the count of 3. Repeat as many times as you can without straining.

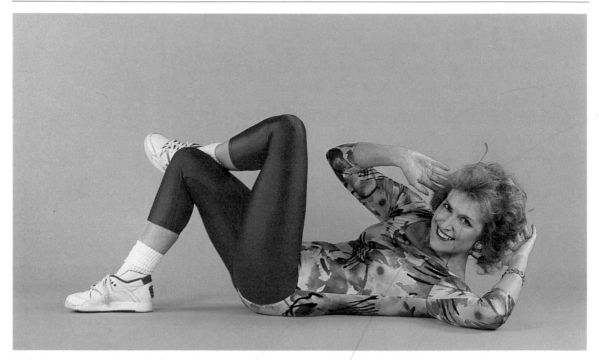

2* Lying on your back on the floor with your knees bent, place your hands to the sides of your head (not at the back). Raise one leg in front of the other. Twist the opposite elbow towards the bent and raised knee. Hold for 2 seconds then return to the floor. Repeat twice more then return the raised leg to the starting position.

Raise the other leg and twist the opposite elbow towards it.

Hold for a count of 2 then return to the floor. Repeat twice more.

Increase the number of repetitions as you become stronger.

*NB Avoid this exercise if your diastasis recti abdominis gap is more than 2 fingers in width. See the Introduction to Postnatal Exercises, page 177.

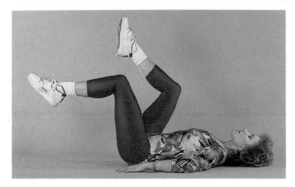

3 Lie on your back on the floor with your hands by your sides. Raise both legs off the floor, keeping your back flat and pushed down into the floor, and cycle in the air. Cycle only for as long as is comfortable. Increase the time spent doing this exercise as you become stronger.

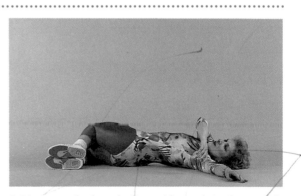

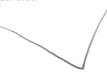

4 Lie on your back on the floor with your knees bent and do this relaxing exercise by gently twisting and stretching your body. Slowly lower your bent knees over to one side as you twist your upper body and arms to the opposite side. Hold for the count of 10 then slowly raise up to the starting position then twist to the other side.

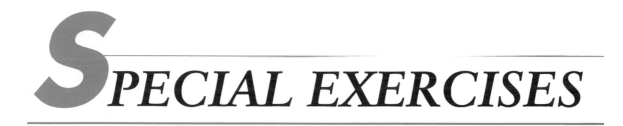

SPECIAL EXERCISES

Whether it be advancing years, a disability, an accident or ailment that has caused you to be physically restricted, there is no reason why you should not attempt to exercise. Everyone's physical ability or disability differs and so our bodies must be worked accordingly to reach the level of which they are capable. On the next few pages you will find a selection of exercises designed to be performed from a chair. Try to do as many as you can. It is just as important for people with restricted mobility to exercise their heart as it is for those who are more physically able. And don't ever think that exercising in a chair is of little benefit. All exercise is relative to the other activities we do in our everyday lives. Working your heart harder, not only improves your general state of health but also your mobility, muscle strength, co-ordination, circulation and, in particular, your morale.

It is always advisable to check with your doctor or specialist before commencing any exercise programme. Exercise should always be progressive and you should never attempt to do too much too soon. Starting off with just a few repetitions of each exercise not only allows our muscles and joints to acclimatise to the movements, it enables our brain to adjust and helps us to develop co-ordination. The more we practise the more we are able to improve our technique and perform the exercises to maximum benefit.

Use your first day's workout simply as a means of familiarising yourself with the movements. On your second day count the repetitions and record the number on the Progress Record Chart. Next time you exercise, attempt to increase the number of repetitions slightly. You'll be surprised and encouraged by your progress. Play some music to improve your momentum.

PROGRESS RECORD CHART

- 1 Swinging arms side to side
- 2 Shoulder rolling
- 3 Alternate shoulder raises
- 4 Spine twists
- 5 Clenching and stretching fingers
- 6 Toe flexing and pointing
- 7 Rolling arms, leaning forwards and reaching up
- 8 Reaching up with both arms
- 9 Raising alternate knees
- 10 Raising both legs out straight
- 11 Alternate elbows to opposite knees
- 12 Alternate elbows to raised opposite knees
- 13 Spine away from chair
- 14 Arm circles
- 15 Clapping

CHAIR EXERCISES

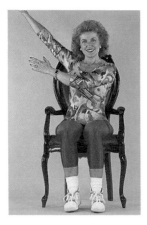

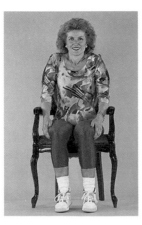

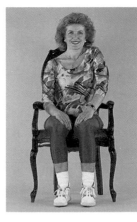

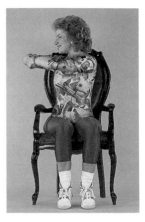

1 Swinging arms side to side
Sit up with a good posture and swing your arms from side to side, making the movement as big as you can. Repeat as many times as possible, according to your fitness and ability.

2 Shoulder rolling
Sit up with a good posture and lean slightly forwards in the chair. Roll your shoulders backwards as many times as you can comfortably. Repeat the movement in a forwards direction.

3 Alternate shoulder raises
Sit up with a good posture and lean slightly forwards in the chair. Raise one shoulder up towards your ear then lower it. Repeat with the other shoulder. Continue for as many repetitions as possible.

Always practise the above 3 warm-up exercises before proceeding.

4 Spine twists
Sit up with a good posture, slightly forwards in the chair. Bend your elbows and place one arm on top of the other in front of you. Slowly twist to each side, pausing in the central position before twisting to the other side. Keep arms as high as possible but not above shoulder level. Do as many twists as is comfortable.

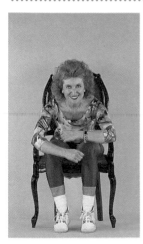

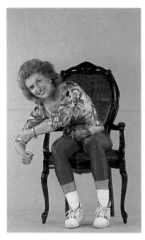

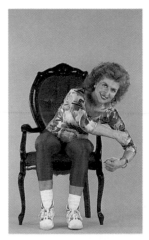

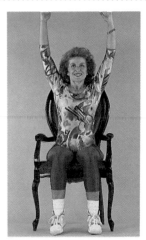

7 Rolling arms, leaning forwards and reaching up
Sitting up in the chair, roll your arms around each other and try leaning forwards, reaching downwards towards your feet with your arms. Slowly

return to the upright position and continue rolling your arms upwards, above your head. Repeat the exercise, this time rolling your arms down to your right side, back to the centre and up above your head,

then down to your left side, back to the centre and up above your head. Repeat the whole sequence 3–5 times, according to your ability.

8 Reaching up with both arms
Sitting up with a good posture, raise both arms towards the ceiling, then slowly lower them. Repeat as many times as you feel is comfortable.

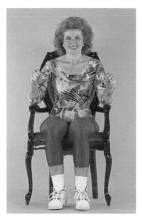

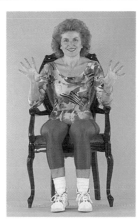

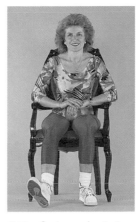

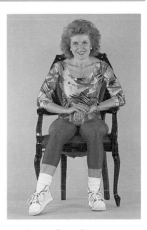

5 Clenching and stretching fingers
Sitting comfortably with a good posture, stretch then clench your fingers. Repeat as many times as is comfortable.

6 Toe flexing and pointing
Sit up with a good posture, slightly forwards in the chair. Point and then flex your toes. Repeat 8 times with one foot then repeat with the other one. Repeat the whole sequence again if you wish.

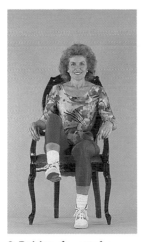

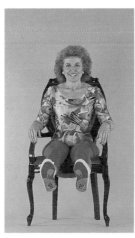

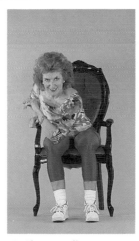

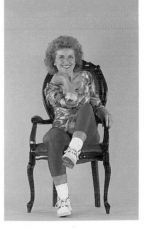

9 Raising alternate knees
Sitting comfortably in the chair, raise one knee then return your foot to the floor or resting point. Repeat with the other knee. Continue raising alternate knees.

10 Raising both legs out straight
Keep your shoulders aligned above your hips (do not lean backwards), raise both legs straight out in front then bend and lower them again.

11 Alternate elbows to opposite knees
Sit up with a good posture and twist your trunk so that one elbow moves towards its opposite knee. Repeat with the other elbow and knee.

12 Alternate elbows to raised opposite knees
Raise one knee and twist your trunk to turn opposite elbow to raised knee. Relax and repeat with the other elbow to the other knee.

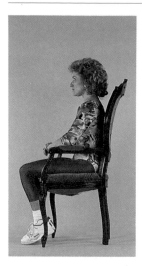

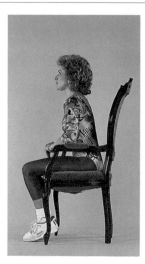

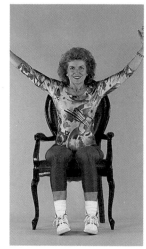

13 Spine away from chair
With your hands relaxed in your lap, just lean forwards and stretch your spine away from the back of the chair.

Relax and repeat. Repeat 10 times to begin with and then increase the number of repetitions, according to your fitness and ability.

14 Arm circles
Sit up with a good posture and move your arms in large circles. Continue for as many repetitions as is comfortable.

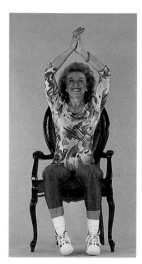

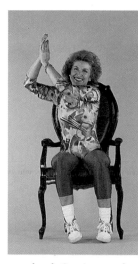

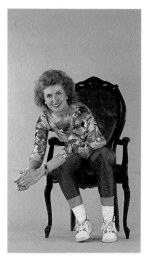

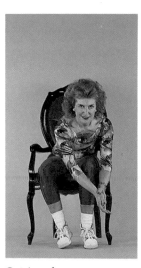

15 Clapping
Sit up with a good posture and clap your hands above

your head. Continue to clap whilst moving your arms in a clockwise direction in a

large circle around your body. Repeat in an anti-clockwise direction.

Continue for as many repetitions as is comfortable.

EXERCISING WITH EQUIPMENT

Exercise machines can be very helpful in our efforts to become fitter and look better and some people do prefer to work out with equipment. Not only can exercise machines enable our body to work our cardiovascular system very hard for long periods of time without placing great strain on our joints (e.g. cycling on a machine rather than jogging), some people find that an external aid to their workout brings a psychological stimulus too.

However, all exercise equipment, whether large or small, relatively cheap or very expensive, will only help you IF YOU USE IT REGULARLY. Before you buy a piece of equipment consider whether you really will use it regularly and where you are going to put it. Second-hand equipment is often available at a fraction of the cost of new equipment, and is often advertised in local newspapers. Alternatively, a range of new equipment, including my own range of equipment, is available from sports outlets.

EXERCISE BIKES

An exercise bike is a useful tool for any family interested in maintaining or increasing their fitness. Most exercise bikes offer different settings so that we can start exercising at a low setting and then, as our body becomes fitter, we can increase the 'gear' resistance as well as the length of time we spend exercising, to help us achieve even greater fitness. Variable settings also mean that each member of the family can exercise at his or her comfortable level.

Cycling provides an excellent aerobic workout. It uses the large muscle groups of the legs and encourages the heart to work hard thus making

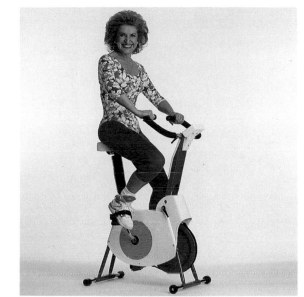

us fitter. Time yourself each time you exercise and record how long you spend cycling and the setting chosen. Increase these as you become fitter. You'll be surprised how quickly regular practice increases your fitness.

However, an exercise bike used only as a clothes-horse will do little for your fitness or your figure. Before buying one, do be certain you will use it regularly.

ROWING MACHINES

Rowing machines offer a most efficient aerobic workout because they exercise both the arms and the legs. Some people who are physically restricted are unable to exercise while standing on their legs so a rowing machine offers an ideal alternative. Some machines (as shown) can be used for other exercises in addition to rowing, to enable you to work a wider range of muscles.

Used regularly, a rowing machine will help to tone you up and make you fitter. It is a good all-

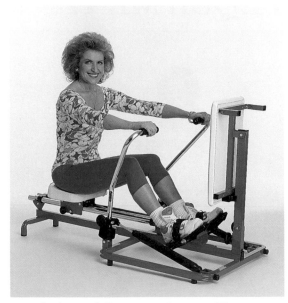

round piece of fitness equipment. However, a rowing machine stored away in the loft will do little except gather dust. Make a realistic assessment of your determination to be fitter and trimmer before buying one.

SKIPPING ROPE

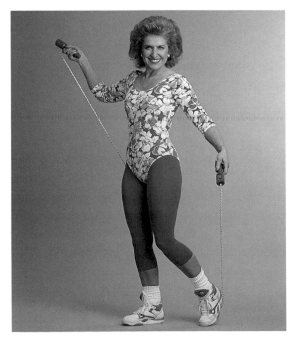

A skipping rope is ideal for an aerobic workout. Buy a skipping rope that is long enough for you to use comfortably. It should just touch the ground when you hold it with outstretched arms. Don't expect to skip for **10** minutes the first time you use your rope. Start with as many skips as you can do without getting too out of breath. You should be able to talk easily while skipping. If not, you are overdoing it, so stop **immediately**.

Keep a record of your progress by recording your increasing number of skips on this chart:

DATE	NO. OF SKIPS

DUMB-BELLS

Commence your workout using the lighter dumb-bells and progress to working with heavier ones only when you feel your body has become used to the lighter ones. It is *important* for your body to acclimatise itself to the use of weights. You will achieve greater benefit with less discomfort by starting gently and increasing the level of weights gradually.

Always stand with your knees slightly bent and your back straight

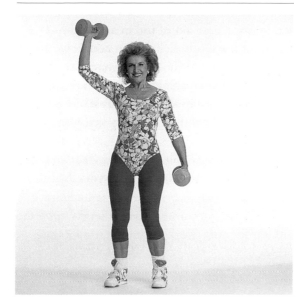

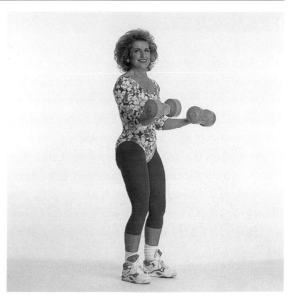

Alternately raise one dumb-bell above your head as you lower the other one.
Repeat 10 times at first, increasing the number of repetitions as you get fitter.

Holding the dumb-bells in front of you, slowly bend then straighten your arms.
Repeat 10 times at first, increasing the number of repetitions as you get fitter.

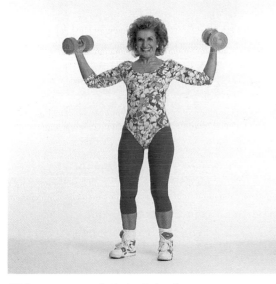

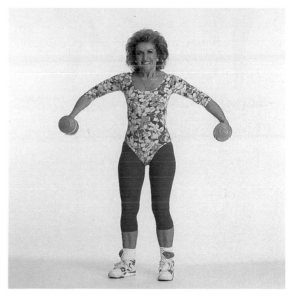

With arms outstretched, slowly bend your arms up towards your head then straighten them again.
Repeat 5 times at first, increasing the number of repetitions as you get fitter.

NB All movements should be controlled and performed slowly. Avoid jerky movements or 'locking' of the joints.

Start with arms outstretched, then bend your arms towards your body and extend them outwards again without slumping forwards.
Repeat 10 times.

TRAMPOLINE

A trampoline is an ideal way to work out aerobically without placing your legs, ankles and feet under excess strain. It is particularly useful for anyone who is overweight. This is because the trampoline acts as a magnificent shock-absorber as we land on the ground. When you realise that after we jump the impact of our body landing on the floor is ten times heavier than normal, it is plain to see that for anyone who is seriously overweight (i.e. 3 stones [19kg] or more) the stress on the joints is enormous and even dangerous. All the aerobic exercises shown in this book which are performed on the spot (in other words, not 'travelling' movements) could be done on a trampoline. Small trampolines (as shown) are not very expensive and can be extremely helpful to some people.

Here are a selection of exercises that will tone up your body while exercising your heart. To make your body work harder, try adding 1 lb (0.5 kg) weights around your wrists (*not* the ankles) for your workout on the trampoline.

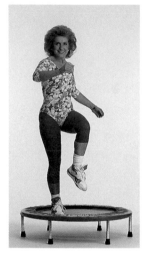

Jogging

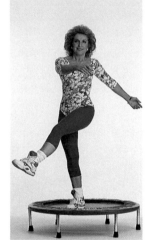

Kicking

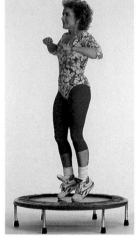

Jumping

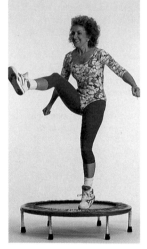

High kicks

INDEX

ROSEMARY CONLEY VIDEOS

The following videos, produced by BBC Video, are available on VHS and can be obtained by mail order from Rosemary Conley Enterprises.

	Quantity	Total Price (£)
Whole Body Programme (approx. 60 minutes) @ £10.99 each	_____	_____
Whole Body Programme II (approx. 60 minutes) @ £10.99 each	_____	_____
The 7–Day Workout (approx. 80 minutes) @ £10.99 each	_____	_____
The Pregnancy and Postnatal Exercise Video [with Jane Ashton] (approx. 90 minutes) @ £10.99 each	_____	_____

TOTAL _____

I enclose a cheque/postal order for £

Please write in BLOCK CAPITALS

NAME: _____
(MR, MRS, MS, MISS)

ADDRESS: _____

_____ POSTCODE: _____

Prices include postage and packing. All cheques should be made payable to Rosemary Conley Enterprises. PLEASE WRITE YOUR NAME AND ADDRESS ON THE REVERSE SIDE OF THE ᵀEQUE AND THE TITLE OF THE VIDEO YOU REQUIRE. Please allow 21 days for delivery. ᵗend your order to: Rosemary Conley Enterprises, P.O. Box 4, Mountsorrel, Loughborough, ᶦʳe LE12 7LB

ᵈetails of the full range of ⁿducts available by mail ʳge, stamped, self- ʳᵉ address. Mark ᵅlogue Request'. ᵘsed volume of work ᵥed, Rosemary Conley

very much regrets that she is not able to reply to readers' letters or problems personally. However, if you have a simple question regarding this or any of her other diets, Rosemary or a member of her very small staff will do their best to answer it, but please keep your letter very brief and enclose a stamped, self-addressed envelope.